Live Your Way Thin

***

Copyright © 2005 Stavros Mastrogiannis
ISBN: 1-4196-1422-3

***

To order additional copies, please contact us.
BookSurge, LLC
www.booksurge.com
1-866-308-6235
orders@booksurge.com

STAVROS MASTROGIANNIS

LIVE YOUR WAY THIN
HOW TO MAKE WEIGHT LOSS INEVITABLE

2005

Live Your Way Thin

CONTENTS

ACKNOWLEDGMENTS

First, I would like to thank the most important person in my life, my wife Svetlana, for her understanding and support while I was writing this book. I worked many long days trying to finish this book, which took away a lot of our time together.

Many people have helped in the creation of my weight loss program **Live Your Way Thin** and in the writing of this book. I would especially like to thank my clients at Olympus Personal Training & Weight Management because without their input and without the trust they put in me, this book would never have been written. I would like to extend a special thanks to Margaret McKay, Wendy Marshall, and Dan Lane who donated a lot of their time to help me develop this program and write this book.

I would also like to thank my family and Barry Miller for their support and help in developing my personal training business, on which my book is based, and also Lisa Sollicito and Jacky Smith for their help with editing this book.

The following people, although I have never met them in person, have had a great impact on my life. Their inspiration through their books and tapes has kept my motivation alive throughout the seemingly endless research that went into developing and writing **Live Your Way Thin**. Thank you, Robert Allen and Anthony Robbins.

HOW THIS PROGRAM CAME ABOUT

Congratulations on your purchase of the **Live Your Way Thin** weight loss program! My name is Stavros Mastrogiannis, and I am the developer of this amazingly effective weight loss system. I hold numerous certifications and a diploma in the fitness, nutrition, and weight management field and I have a degree in Culinary Arts, from the Culinary Institute of America. I have been in the fitness and weight management field for over 12 years and I would like to share with you how I came up with this weight loss system. I love what I do, and I know my program can help anyone who needs to lose weight and is willing to put in some effort. The only people who will not lose weight on my program are those who have medical problems that prevent them from losing weight. However, even for these people this program will have health benefits. (As an aside, less than 2% of the obesity cases in the United States are due to medical problems) Therefore, the chances are that this program will work for you. However, I always advise people to check with their doctor before starting any weight loss program.

When people ask me what kind of work I do, I tell them that I don't work; I practice my passion: helping people achieve their dream of a lean and healthy body of which they can be proud. There is nothing more satisfying than helping people who are overweight, unfit, and unhappy with their bodies achieve the body of their dreams. They truly get a new lease on life. Their posture changes, their faces glow, and their mental attitude changes. They become a completely new person. No matter how many times I have seen a client transform like this, it is always a great feeling and I share in their happiness.

However, things were not always this satisfying. When I first began in this field, I faced some frustrating years. Although I was applying all the information I had learned through my schooling, I was still unable to help many of my clients lose the weight they wanted. Take Shari, for example. She worked diligently, yet she was not losing weight and she was not getting the lean body she deserved. She felt frustrated and discouraged, and my heart went out to her. I vowed I would find the secrets that would work for her and for other clients, too. During those years, I learned many important lessons, and one of the most important was that there is a lot more to losing weight and getting in shape than what they taught me at school. This is when I opened my mind to other possibilities and started doing my own research. I started reading anything I could get my hands on that had to do with weight loss, exercise, and motivation. I subscribed to many newsletters and other health related publications, including those from The John Hopkins Medical Institute, the University of California at Berkeley, and the Mayo Clinic. I also started observing how people who were in good shape stayed that way. As a Greek-American, I traveled to Greece and other European nations quite often and noticed many tended to have thinner populations. I observed what they ate and how their physical activities varied. I also remembered when I was living in Greece and going to school, they were very few kinds over weight. I would say out of 350 kids that were in my, school maybe three or four were overweight. I remembered how our diet in Greece was so much different from here in the United States and how much more active people were, both young and old. Then I began to add some of these elements to programs for my clients.

As my approach evolved, something wonderful happened: more and more of my clients began to see results. I was amazed, because on the surface my approach was very simple. There was no crazy diet or overly strenuous exercise program. What I discovered was that there are four crucial ingredients to losing weight and building a lean and healthy body, and when those four ingredients are incorporated into someone's life, a lean and healthy body is inevitable. Now I am in the great position of being able to help the vast majority of my clients achieve the body they want, and it is a great feeling.

I am so excited about my discovery that I want to share it with the world so everybody can experience the great feeling and great energy that comes with achieving the body of your dreams, a body that you can be proud to call your own, just like my clients have been experiencing at my gym. Because not everyone can come to Danbury and work out individually with me at my gym, I have recreated it in a book form and

I called it **Live Your Way Thin**. Now many more people can get the same information that has worked for my clients, and it can work for you, too.

Sincerely,
Stavros Mastrogiannis

P.S. I always like to get feedback from people that try my weight loss system. Feel free to email me with any comments and/or success stories you have. You can email me at: Stavros@StavrosM.com

INTRODUCTION

There are numerous fitness gurus out there, with fancy books and videotapes that claim their product is the only thing you need to lose weight and get in shape. In doing research for this program, I read many of these books and watched many of the tapes, learning as I went along. I subscribe to many excellent fitness and health newsletters and magazines including ACSM's Health & Fitness Journal, Mayo Clinic Health Letter, University of California, Berkeley Wellness Letter, IDEA Personal Trainer, IDEA Health & Fitness Source, and Health Club Products Review, and these subscriptions have provided me with a wealth of helpful information. But do you know where I learned the most? Working with my clients and actually trying different exercise programs and different diets, seeing what works in real life and what does not. Figuring out what really motivates people to exercise, what the best way is to incorporate exercise and proper nutrition into a real person's life—someone who has a job and a family to consider when making a lifestyle change—is a challenge. Just because something works in a lab does not mean it will work in real life.

I have found three major problems with most diet and exercise programs on the market these days. First, they are not very healthy! Yes, on most diets, people will lose weight if the diet is followed correctly. The problem is a lot of the diets do not provide all the nutrients your body needs to maintain good health and you cannot stay on them long term. The second problem with all the weight loss programs, at least the ones I have seen, is that they have you make big changes in your eating and activity habits overnight. Although in many programs you do lose weight, very few people can sustain the weight loss because very few people can change that quickly and be able to adapt the new changes into their life. That is why the vast majority of people eventually go back to their old habits and gain back all the weight, and in many cases even more. The third problem is incomplete information! Let me first give you one fact that no weight loss expert can dispute. There are four keys to losing weight and keeping it off long term, and you need to incorporate all four keys in order to succeed. The four keys are:

1) Cardiovascular Training (Aerobics), 2) Resistance Training, 3) Proper Nutrition, and 4) Consistency. All the books I have read and all the tapes I have watched only tell you about one or two of the four keys. This could explain why, although there are so many books out there on weight loss and health, the weight of the average American is still going up at a rate of one to two pounds per year. If you do not believe me, look at the article that was written in USA TODAY in section D, on Thursday, May 8, 2004. The books and tapes only give you part of the solution to your weight loss problem. Don't get me wrong—I am not saying that all diet and exercise books out there are bad; on the contrary, some of them are very good, but they only give you one piece of the puzzle, and you still need three more. Even if you have all the pieces, you still need to learn how to fit them into your life. This is where **Live Your Way Thin** comes in. **Live Your Way Thin** is the only weight loss program, to my knowledge, that covers all four keys and shows you how to incorporate them into your life and into your daily habits. The only way to lose weight permanently is through your daily habits. All the information in this program is based on facts and well-based theories, but most importantly has been tried and tested on my clients with great results. If you are looking for a temporary quick-fix solution to your weight problem, this is not the program for you. If, on the other hand, you want to lose weight the right way once and for all and improve your health in the process, this is the program for you. Just like my clients, most people do not have time to waste. For this reason, I have kept the book short with only the essential information you need to succeed. I have broken down the whole program into four simple steps; all you have to do is follow the steps one at a time, complete each step and than move to the next one. Each step builds on the previous one and there is no time limit on how long you have to stay on each step. The only people that might not see results are those who have a medical condition that prevents them from losing weight. I suggest that before starting any exercise or weight loss program, you consult your doctor.

I am very excited to introduce **Live Your Way Thin** to the world and I truly believe that **Live Your Way Thin** is the beginning of the end for excess weight and obesity. For the latest updates on weight loss or upcoming seminars in your area, please visit out my web site, <u>www. StavrosM.com</u>.

CHAPTER 1

We Have a Weight Problem

Nobody was meant to be fat.

Allow me to let you in on this secret: although some people have the tendency to gain weight easily due to genetic factors, even those people would not gain weight if they ate the way nature intended them to eat and maintained an active lifestyle, because the human body was built to be active. Less than 2% of all cases of obesity are due to medical reasons. The main reason why people are overweight is not due to bad genes but to bad eating habits and inactivity, and both are under our complete control. I am telling you this because what you believe has a great effect on what you can achieve. Nobody was meant to be fat; our bad habits got us there.

One major reason why people cannot lose weight and achieve the body of their dreams is that they have never truly believed they could do it in the first place. Many people believe they were meant to be fat by nature and they blame their bad genes for the body they have. I am here to prove these people wrong. Nature's design was for all humans to have a fit body. Do you think nature intended for some people to be overweight or obese? I don't think so, because if it did, why are only humans overweight and not other mammals? You do not see overweight lions or deer. One reason is that humans are the only mammals that have denaturized their food. Wild animals eat the way nature intended them to eat and their bodies have adapted to handling that food. Modern humans, on the other hand, eat differently than the way nature intended them to eat; the human body could not handle the new denaturized food and as a result, there are many overweight and obese people. In addition to this, we are also suffering from many degenerative diseases that are literally killing us. Even our pets, whose diets we control, suffer from many of the same diseases.

The human body was build to be active. To prove this, let me ask you a question. What happens to the human body when it is not active? It atrophies! The muscles become smaller and weaker; the bones lose density; the heart becomes weaker; the lungs lower their ability to extract oxygen from the air breathed in; and the blood lowers the amount of oxygen it can deliver to the muscles and organs. As the body atrophies, the amount of energy it needs to sustain itself goes down. These are only a few of the many things that happen to the human body when it is not active. Active, by the way, does not necessarily mean exercising. To sum up: we eat a highly denaturized diet with a lot of empty calories (calories that provide no nutritional value such as junk food), and we are the least active we have ever been due to all the modern conveniences. It is no wonder that so many people cannot maintain the fit look their body was meant to have by design.

If you are ready to get your body looking and feeling the way it was meant to, read on.

America is gaining weight year after year. WHY?

In America, we spend $34 billion per year on weight loss products and we are still gaining weight at the rate of one to two pounds per year on average. Sixty-one percent of Americans are overweight or obese and the numbers are rising. With weight gain and an increase in body fat comes many other health problems like heart disease (the #1 killer in America), stroke, diabetes, and some forms of cancer to name but a few. Obesity is costing this country $100 billion each year. We had better start doing something about this because it will only get worse. However, it would appear that we are doing something about it. After all, are we not spending $34 billion per year on weight loss products? Well, many of the weight loss products on the market are part of the problem, but that is a whole other story, which I will cover later. Now let us examine the main factors that contribute to the weight gain problem. **Understanding the problem is the first step to finding a solution.**

Factor #1 We eat more.

The average American eats around 300 to 500 calories per day more than they did 30 years ago. One national survey found that adults underestimate their daily caloric intake, on average, by about 800 calories. We are eating calories we don't even know we are eating. Eating has become such a habit for some people that they eat without even knowing it, as if they are on autopilot. Many of my clients, when asked if they eat too much, tell me, "Oh no, I don't eat that much," but when I ask them to keep a food journal, they realize they eat a lot more than they thought.

Factor #2 We eat the wrong food.

On average, we consume the equivalent of 34 teaspoons of added sugar every day. Here we have around 500 calories from sugar alone. This sugar comes from all the sweets we eat and sodas we drink. There is also a lot of added sugar that we are not even aware of in processed food. In addition to this, the consumption of grain products has gone up 50% in the last 30 years. Unfortunately, it is refined grain products such as white bread, pasta, and snack chips that we are eating.

I worked in the restaurant business for many years and I have seen with my own eyes how and what people eat. I would like to tell you one of many experiences I had. I was working at a catering hall, at a wedding of around 400 people. The menu consisted of four courses: a fresh fruit salad, a salad, a main course, and a dessert. The main course was lobster tail and filet mignon, with mashed potato and broccoli. These are my own observations. Some people did not even touch their fruit salad. The same thing was true of the regular salad. When it came to the main course, everybody ate the filet mignon and some people even had seconds; most people ate their lobster tails; and everybody ate their mashed potatoes. But guess what-hardly anyone touched the broccoli. Of course, mostly everyone ate the dessert. The food considered healthy and good for you was hardly eaten, but the meat, potatoes, and of course, the desserts were devoured. For me, this meal summed up why we have a weight problem in America.

Factor #3 We eat for the wrong reasons.

Nowadays people eat for a variety of reasons other than real physical hunger. For example, how many of you go to the movie theater and have a popcorn and a soda even though you have just eaten dinner? How many of you, even though you are not hungry, will still pick on food if it is put in front of you? How many of you will finish everything on your plate even though you are already full? How many times do you finish dinner and although you are completely full, you still have dessert? What has happened is that we do not see food as fuel for the body anymore, but as entertainment-something that will make us feel better, something to do when we are bored, and many other things except what it really is, fuel for the body.

Factor #4 We are less active.

It is estimated that the average person burns around 300 calories less per day than they did 30 years ago. I have even heard estimates that the average person burns 500 to 700 calories less per day than they did 50 years ago. No one really knows for sure how many less calories we burn today than we did 30 to 50 years ago but one thing is certain, we are burning a lot less. Let us think about this. Due to all the modern conveniences, people today do a lot less physical labor than people 30 and 50 years ago. People nowadays watch a lot more television. Do you know how many calories you burn watching television? Not much more than sleeping, especially now that we have remote controls and do not have to get up for anything. Next thing you know, we will have robots bring our food, so we will not have to get up from the couch at all! I have seen people getting into their car, driving to the end of their driveway to pick up the mail, and driving back to their house. How many people have you seen driving around the parking lot at the mall trying to find the closest parking spot? Look at our children. Children years ago were a lot more active than they are today. Children 50 years ago used to play outside running and doing sports. Today children play video games and watch TV indoors. I could write a whole book just on how we have become less active over the years. I believe these examples emphasize just that.

These are the four main factors that I believe have contributed to our weight gain in this country, and many other countries that are following our example. So knowing the factors that contribute to our weight gain, why haven't we been able to lose weight? This is a very good question, which I am going to address next.

Why we haven't been able to lose weight.

There are three main reasons why we haven't been able to lose weight.
- Misinformation
- Habit
- Desire for instant gratification

Misinformation:

I believe this is the main reason why we have not been able to lose weight in America. Unfortunately, most of the $34 billion we spend on weight loss is spent on products that don't work and just help spread the abundance of misinformation that is out there, or products that offer only part of the solution but claim they are the complete solution, which again spreads misinformation. Let me explain.

How many of you have seen the infomercials for ab machines? What do they tell you? They tell you they are perfect for people that need to lose fat from their midsection. They show models with perfect abs; they persuade you that if you use their machine you are going to get abs just like the model and guarantee that you will lose one to two inches in the first two weeks. Well, let me give you some facts. First, the reason you lose one to two inches in the first few weeks is not that you have lost fat, but that your ab muscles have pulled into a straight line. Crunches and all other midsection exercises have absolutely no effect on the fat that you might have on your midsection. In other words, just because you are using your abs does not mean you are losing fat off the abs. There have been plenty of studies to prove that. How many of you have a lot of fat on your legs and have been instructed to do a lot of leg exercises so you can tone them up? Doing leg exercises does not mean you are burning the fat off your legs. What muscle you work has nothing to do with where the fat you are burning will come from. Just because you are using the treadmill does not mean you are burning fat only from your legs. You cannot spot reduce. Your genetic make-up determines from where the fat is burned, not the type of exercise you do. This is only an example of the misinformation the public is fed.

Other infomercials advertising aerobic machines tell you that they are all you need to lose weight and get in shape. Again, WRONG! Aerobic exercise, although very important, is only part of the solution. You still need to do some form of resistance training and eat a proper diet, but of course you are not told this and if you are, it is in fine print at the bottom of the screen. Again, the public is misinformed.

A prime example of misinformation is diet pills. They put people on TV telling you that they lost 20, 30, 40 pounds in one month using whatever diet pill they are advertising, and of course at the bottom of the screen in fine print is written, 'results not typical.' Of course results are not typical because the people you see on TV are the exceptions. We do not know what else they did other than taking those pills. They could be watching their diet and exercising. Many diet pill manufacturers recommend diet and exercise as you are taking the pills. Take 1000 people, give them any pill and a decent exercise and diet program, and you will always have one or two that will lose a lot of weight. These people are the exceptions, but unfortunately, they are the people you see on TV. This is why they have to put a disclaimer at the bottom of the screen. The problem is, many people see these commercials and think losing five to ten pounds per week is normal, so when they start a weight loss program and only lose one to two pounds per week, which is the norm, they feel like failures and they quit.

Another great example of misinformation in the fitness field is that you must do three sets per exercise to get results. I heard this often in the gyms where I worked. People spend one to two hours in the gym weight training because they believe this is what they must do to get results. Did you know that if you are a beginner who has never lifted weight before or has not lifted weights in a long time, there is no difference in muscle or strength gain, between doing one set per exercise or three sets per exercise? The only difference is that when you do three sets it will take you three times longer to get your workout done. If weight loss is your goal, instead of spending all that extra time weight training, do aerobics or plan your meals, both of which would be of great benefit to your weight-loss efforts. These are just few examples of how misinformed we are about losing weight and getting in shape.

We are creatures of habit.

Besides being misinformed about how to lose weight, most weight loss programs do not fully address how to break old habits and develop new ones. Most weight loss programs focus on the short term and, even if you lose weight, you cannot sustain it long term. The high protein diets are one of the best examples. I personally know quite a few people who have lost weight on a high protein diet and gained it all back, in some cases even more. In fact, I do not know of anyone who has kept all the weight off more than one year. Your current habits, good or bad, are responsible for the shape you are in today. Only by changing your habits will you be able to make permanent changes to your shape and your weight. Changing a habit requires initial effort, but the good news is that it usually takes about 21 days to start developing a new habit. Therefore, in the beginning, you might have to will yourself to take the new actions until they become habits. Although there are mental exercises that I will be covering in this program that will make developing new habits much easier, you still have to do them. There is no way around this. You see very few weight loss programs explain to people that it will take some initial effort to get in shape. Unfortunately, many of the weight loss products you see on the market today have only one purpose, and that is to make lots of money for the people that own them. They will tell people whatever they want to hear just as long as they buy the product. This goes back to misinformation. It is unfortunate that they have found loopholes in consumer protection laws that allow them to get away with all the misinformation they are spreading.

Instant Gratification

Most people these days want and expect instant gratification, and this is a big problem in the weight loss industry. People want to start a weight loss program today and lose the weight by tomorrow. Unfortunately, many unethical companies tell people whatever they want to hear as long as they buy their product, instead of telling people the truth about losing weight and how fast they should expect to lose the weight. They make promises such as, "You can have the body you want in six weeks or less.", "Lose 30 pounds in 30 days.", "Lose two inches in one week.", etc. All these promises play on the fact that people are looking for instant gratification.

The question is, how can you promise anyone that they can have the body they want in six weeks or less when you do not know their current weight? Are they telling me that if I was 100 pounds overweight I would be able to have the body I want in six weeks? I highly doubt it. The Atkins diet and other high protein diets have caught on because of people's drive for instant gratification. Yes, I would agree that with those diets, most people lose weight quickly, but my question is, at what cost?

Unfortunately, many people want to lose weight so badly that will try anything as long as they lose weight quickly, without taking into consideration the future consequences. The high protein craze is still fairly new, and we do not fully know all the effects this diet has on the human body. One thing for certain is that all the people I know who have done a high protein diet have lost weight, but did not feel that great while on the diet; all of them have regained the weight because they could not sustain the diet. What is the point of losing weight if you are going to gain it all back anyway, and what is the point of being thin if you are weak and lethargic? More and more studies are showing the dangers of a high protein diet and most weight loss experts, including myself, would advise against it. You are far better off losing the weight slowly, the healthy way. The average person following a healthy weight loss program will lose around one to two pounds per week. Of course, there are exceptions. I have seen people lose between five and seven pounds per week, but as I said, those people are the exceptions. You can take 100 people, give them the same weight loss program, and you will have one or two that will lose weight very quickly. These people are the ones you see on the weight loss commercials, and this is why they have to put in fine print at the bottom of the screen, "Results not typical." or "Results may vary." They are also the people appearing on talk shows to talk about any particular diet. The problem with this is that people see the commercials and the talk shows and think losing five to ten pounds a week is normal, so when they lose only one to two pounds per week they feel discouraged and stop. The truth is, there are no shortcuts to fitness; there is no magic pill that makes weight come off instantly. If there were one, everybody would be thin and fit by now. The fact is, you will need to put some effort into it. Here is something no weight loss program will ever tell you, but they should, because doing this will greatly improve your chances of keeping the weight off for life. When you first start a weight loss program, your goal for the first three or four weeks is not to lose weight, but to start establishing the right eating and exercise habits. Any weight loss at this point is bonus. Once you have established a good routine and you have started to get used to it, you can start pushing yourself and you will start to see results. Doing it this way gives your body and mind a chance to adapt to the new changes. Unfortunately, no weight loss program I have ever seen will tell you this, and that is why most of them fail. However, there is some good news. There is instant gratification from doing it this way. You will start feeling better, stronger, and more energetic within the first three weeks of your weight loss program. So if the weight is not coming off fast enough for you, think of how much better you feel; how you are improving your health; how you are lowering the risk of developing many degenerative diseases; and best of all by doing it my way, the results are more likely to stick. The other good news is that the first three weeks are always the hardest; once you get past the first three weeks the new actions start becoming habits and it is a much easier ride after that. So remember, do not fall victim to commercials that play on your desire for instant gratification. Now you know the truth.

CHAPTER 2

The Solution to our Weight Problem

The complete solution to your weight problem.

In the previous chapter, we covered all the factors that are preventing us from losing weight. In this chapter, we are going to talk about the solution to the problem. If you are willing to follow my recommendations and put a little effort into it, weight loss and good health is inevitable. First, I would like to explain to you the four keys to losing weight, and in the next chapter, I will help you put your weight loss program together.

The four Keys to weight loss

As you know, there are many different and conflicting opinions when it comes to losing weight and getting in shape. Let me give you a **fact** that no one can argue with: there are four keys to losing weight and building a lean, healthy body: **Key #1** Resistance training; **Key #2** Cardiovascular training (Aerobics); **Key #3** Proper Nutrition (not just what you eat but when and how you eat); **Key #4** Consistency. Take one away and you have failure. You might be able to lose some weight but you will not be as healthy and you will not be able to keep the weight off long term. What is the point of losing weight if you cannot keep it off? If somebody can argue on this fact they should not be in the weight loss business, because they do not know all the facts.

Now, as I told you before, it will take some effort to achieve your goals. Nothing worthwhile comes without effort. You have spent many years building your current lifestyle habits. Change will not be quick and easy, but it can happen if you want it to happen.

The good news is that if you lose weight and get in shape the right way, it does become easier and even fun over time. The best way to lose body fat and keep it off for life is by developing healthy, lifelong habits. Do that and you will keep the weight off for the rest of your life. If you have to keep putting forth great effort at keeping the weight off, as is the case with most diets, eventually you will get tired and give up. I would give up too. A habit is something you do without thinking. This is what this weight loss program is all about, replacing your unhealthy lifestyle habits with healthy, fat-burning lifestyle habits.

The benefits of this program are reduction of body fat, a more toned and healthier looking body, better health, more energy, and much more. Once you achieve your fitness goal, you will be able to maintain the results. As far as effort goes, yes, it will take effort, but it will be like pushing a car from a dead stop. Initially, it will take a lot of effort to get the car to start moving but once it is moving it will be easier to keep pushing. Do not worry, your exercise program will not involve pushing a car!

***

Key # 1—RESISTANCE TRAINING

Resistance training is one of the most neglected parts of a weight loss program. Many misinformed people consider it even less important when it comes to weight loss. Not doing some form of resistance training is a great way to sabotage your results. Resistance training is as important as aerobics and diet if you want to lose weight and keep it off, and do not let anyone tell you otherwise.

Let me explain why: your body is burning calories at all times, even when you are not doing anything. This is your resting metabolic rate. Some people have a higher resting metabolic rate, which means they are burning more calories even at rest. Some people have a lower resting metabolic rate, which means they are burning less calories at rest. One of the factors that determine your resting metabolic rate is the amount of muscle you have. In other words, the more muscle you have, the more calories you burn. One pound of muscle burns up to 35 calories a day in its resting state. Let's say you start doing resistance training and you gain four pounds of muscle; this means you will be burning an extra 140 calories per day, and this is in a resting state. You can lose an extra 14 pounds of fat in a year by simply gaining four pounds of muscle. If you become active by doing aerobics, having more muscle means you will burn more calories.

Let me give you an example. Take two people, one with more muscle than the other, and have them run the same distance at the same pace. The person with the greater muscle mass will burn more calories doing the same activity at the same intensity than the person with less muscle mass. Having more muscle greatly enhances your ability to burn fat. Studies have shown that when you try to lose weight by diet and aerobics alone, 25% of the weight you lose will be muscle. When you lose muscle, you slow down your metabolic rate. This is why, in diet programs that do not include resistance training, despite an initial weight loss, you will hit a plateau. In order to keep losing weight you will need to further reduce your calories. Even if you lose all the weight you want, because of the amount of muscle you have lost, your metabolic rate will have slowed down so much that as soon as you start eating normally you will regain all the weight. Did you know that less than 2% of the people who lose weight by diet alone are able to keep the weight off long term? Even if you are not trying to lose weight, it is important to know that on average, a person who does not do any resistance training loses four pounds of muscle every 10 years. This means that your metabolic rate is slowing down. This is one reason why as you age you gain body fat, even though you continue eating the same amount of food.

One quick note here, most women do not have to worry about bulking up unless they are taking steroids, which I do not recommend.

One of the best and most effective ways to build muscle and tone up is high-intensity strength training. It is only 20 to 30 minutes long and you will only need to do it two times a week. I will be giving you more details on how to do this type of training in Chapter 4. Of course, if you are a beginner, you should never start with the high-intensity strength-training right away. You need to do the beginner's strength training for at least three to four weeks before you start with the high-intensity strength training. This gives your body a chance to adapt to the increased stresses of the high-intensity training. You will find more details on how to start a weight training routine and how to progress in chapter 4.

How much resistance should I use for my resistance training?

When you first start doing resistance training start light, whether you are using weights, machines, or tubing. Your main concern in the first few weeks of resistance training should be getting the form right. Give yourself one to two weeks of light resistance to make sure you have learned the exercises and your muscles have learned the correct path of motion (form). I see too many men and women in the gym lifting a lot of weight incorrectly. What happens is that when they first started to weight train, they concentrated on the amount of weight they could lift and they did not learn proper form. The problem with not having proper form when you lift weight or perform some type of resistance exercise, is that you greatly increase the risk of injury. There is usually more wear and tear on your joints, and in the long run can that manifest itself as an injury. Because this type of injury takes a long time to develop, people don't associate it with their bad form. Their thinking is, "I have been doing this exercise this way for years and it never hurt before!"

Also by having bad form, you do not work the target muscle as effectively as you could. These are only a few of the problems with having bad form. Once you feel you have the form right, then and only then should you start pushing the weights up. You should use enough weight, or whatever type of resistance you are using, so that you can do the number of reps you have chosen to do, with the last two to three reps being so hard that sometimes you are unable to complete the last one. If you can do all the reps with relative ease, it is time to increase the weight. Try to increase the weight in increments of three to five pounds. Go to Chapter 5 for detailed demonstrations of the exercises.

How many sets and how many repetitions should I do?

This depends on what type of training you are doing. For more information, please read Chapter 4.

A summary of what you must know about Resistance Training:

1. If you are new to weight training, start with the beginner's workout. Stay at the beginner's workout for at least three to four weeks before you move up.

2.   With the exception of the first one to two weeks of weight training, when you should keep the weight light and concentrate on form, the weight should be heavy enough so the last two reps of each set are very challenging.

3.   Keep in mind that you need to work out each body part at least two times per week in order to make gains. One time per week is enough to maintain the gains you have made up to that point. Therefore, if you are doing a full body workout, which I would advise you do if you just want to tone up, you should do at least two workouts per week but no more than three, skipping one day between workouts.

4.   If you are trying to lose weight off your legs, doing more leg exercises will not help. In fact if you have bulky legs and you just want to slim them down, I would strongly advise you to do only one compound exercise for your legs, such as Leg Press, Squats or Lunges. A compound exercise will involve most if not all the muscles in your legs and that is enough to tone the leg muscles. Remember, you cannot spot reduce, so doing more leg exercises will not help you lose fat off your legs. The only thing you can accomplish by doing more leg exercises is to bulk up your legs. If that is your goal, then go ahead and do it. Many people, even personal trainers, make this mistake. I do not blame people for making that mistake, especially with all the misleading commercials you see on TV: women with perfect bodies advertising exercising machines that have nothing to do with their physical shape. As far as personal trainers go, they should know better. You have to follow all four keys in order to lose weight. You have absolutely no control over where you will lose the fat; only your genetics do.

5.   You might feel sore after the first few workouts, which is normal, but don't think that if you are not sore you are not getting results. As long as you are doing your workouts properly and you follow the above rules, you are getting results. If you feel sharp pain in your joints or muscles, that is not good. If the pain does not go away consult your doctor.

Key # 2—AEROBIC EXERCISE

First, let us define aerobic exercise. Aerobic exercise is any exercise that requires oxygen for the production of energy. The reason aerobic exercise is important to a weight loss program is that it is the fastest way to burn fat and the fastest way to improve your cardiovascular system, which is very important to overall health and well-being. Moreover, by improving your cardiovascular system, you become more aerobically fit and your body is better able to burn your stored fat, which makes you a better fat-burning machine. Keep in mind that even though you get great benefits from aerobics, it is only one of the four keys you need for successful weight loss. Just doing aerobics without doing anything else can actually sabotage your progress. For example, you can be doing plenty of aerobics and still gain weight because you are not watching your diet. Or did you know that if you are trying to lose weight by doing aerobics only, up to 25% of the weight you will lose will come from muscle, and as you learned in Key #1, Resistance Training, maintaining and/or increasing the muscle you have is very important to a weight loss program. Therefore, the bottom line is that aerobics will help you lose fat but aerobics by themselves can sabotage your weight loss by decreasing your muscle mass. Also, try to stretch after each workout so you prevent the muscles from stiffening up. You can stretch as often as you want but try to stretch at least once per day, holding each stretch for at least 15 seconds or more. The following are examples of indoor and outdoor aerobic exercises you can do. **Outdoors:** Walking, jog, cycle, cross-country ski, hike swim, in-line skate, row. **Indoors:** Treadmill, stair-stepper, stationary cycle, Nordic Track, rowing machine, swim, aerobic classes.

How intense should your cardiovascular workout be?

Research shows that in order to improve your cardiovascular fitness, the best intensity to do aerobics at is 60% to 90% of your maximum heart rate for a minimum of 20 minutes, three times per week, every other day. At what intensity you should do your aerobics depends on your current fitness level. The better cardiovascular shape you are in, the higher the intensity your workout should be; the lower your cardiovascular fitness, the lower the intensity of your workout. People who are greatly out of shape can improve their cardiovascular fitness even with a workout intensity at 50% of their maximum heart rate.

Note the above intensities are to improve your cardiovascular fitness and to maximize fat burning. For fat loss purposes, any aerobic activity, even at a low intensity below 50%, is still better than none and still helps you to lose fat. Ideally, you will want to work out at a higher intensity because you would burn more fat in the same time spent doing the activity, but don't forget you have to take into consideration your current fitness level, how overweight you are, and your age. If you are out of shape, start slowly and work your way up. You always want to work out at the highest intensity you can for your current fitness level, because, as well as burning more over all calories during the workout, your metabolic rate will also stay higher longer after the work out.

If you have heard of the Fat Burning Zone (the intensity at which your body burns fat more efficiently), ignore it. You are always better off working out at the highest intensity your current fitness level allows..

To figure out your maximum heart rate take 220—your age = your maximum heart rate.

(This is an estimate.)

To figure out your target heart rate take 220—your age—Resting Heart Rate (RHR) x the percent you want to workout at + your RHR = your target heart rate. For example, let's say you are 44 years old, a beginner with a RHR of 70. You want to work out between at an intensity level 60% and 70% of your maximum heart rate. This is how to figure it out:

220—44 = 176 (Estimated maximum heart rate)
176—70(RHR) = 106
106 x .60 = 63.60
63.60 +70 = 133.6, round it to 134 beats per minute (bpm)

134 bpm is the heart rate for 60% of your maximum heart rate if you were 44 years old. To work out 70%, follow the same formula.
176—70 = 106
106 x .7 = 74.2
74.2 + 70 = 144.2, round it to 144 bpm.

If you want to work out between 60% and 70% of your maximum heart rate, your heart rate should be between 134 and 144 beats per minute (bpm).

To figure out your heart rate you can take your pulse for 10 seconds and whatever number you get x 6 = your heart rate per minute. An easier way to do it is to get a heart rate monitor; they start at $89. I find heart rate monitors a great motivational tool. Most people find it very hard to keep aerobics at the right intensity, especially when you are a beginner. You can set the heart rate monitor with the maximum and minimum heart rates you would like to stay between, so when your heart rate goes over or under the preset heart rate, an alarm goes off and you know to speed up or slow down in order to stay within your target heart rate range. The benefit of having a heart rate monitor is motivation. It helps some people push themselves to staying in their target heart rate zone. If you take the time to do aerobics, you might as well get the most out of it, and a heart rate monitor helps you do just that.

Although using a heart rate monitor is a great idea if you want to spend the money to get one, what I have found works the best as far as motivating yourself to push harder and keeping up the intensity of the workout is to keep track of the number of calories you burn per workout in a set amount of time. In other words, let's say you ran on the treadmill and you burned 100 calories in 30 minutes. Next time you do the treadmill, try to burn more calories in the same amount of time. By having a goal to reach on each aerobic workout, you will find it easier to push yourself to reach that goal. Of course, you must use the same aerobic machine because each aerobic machine is calibrated differently and the calorie count from machine to machine is not necessarily. If you are running outside, then keep track of the amount of time it takes you to cover a particular path. Each time, try to cover the same path in a shorter time.

Note: If you are a healthy individual with no heart condition, are not pregnant, and have no doctor's restrictions, don't worry if your heart rate is over your upper heart rate limit as long as you are feeling OK. The estimated heart rate zone can be off by up to 20 beats. The key here is that you are feeling OK during your workout.

Other ways to measure aerobic intensity without taking your heart rate is the talk test. Although not as accurate as taking your heart rate, it is still a good indicator of intensity.

When you work out aerobically you should be able to talk, but you should not be able to sing. If you want to increase the intensity, then you should be able to talk but not very comfortably. If you cannot talk at all, then the workout is too intense and you should slow down.

If you choose not to use heart rate to measure the intensity of an aerobic workout, use the following rating system. **Warning! This system does not measure intensity of an aerobic workout as accurately as measuring your heart rate but it does give you an idea. If you have any cardiovascular problems or you are pregnant and your doctor has given you a specific heart rate zone he/she wants you to stay within, then use a heart rate monitor to measure your heart rate more accurately.**

Ratings:

Very Low (VL) example: a very slow walk. Low (L) example: walking. Medium (M) example: fast-paced walking. Medium High (MH) example: a very fast walk or slow jog. High (H) example: a jog to fast jog. Very High (VH) example: running or sprinting.

***

A summary of what you must know about Cardiovascular Exercises (Aerobics):

1. The minimum you can do and still improve your cardiovascular fitness is 20 minutes, three times per week at an intensity you find somewhat challenging. Keep in mind that for weight loss purposes, any aerobics is helpful.

2. When you are doing aerobics to lose weight, don't worry as much about range of heart rate, unless of course of you have a heart condition or you are pregnant and have strict instructions from your doctor not to exceed a particular heart rate. Your estimated maximum heart rate can be off by as much as 20 beats, which makes any calculations that use your estimated maximum heart rate reasonably inaccurate. The best thing you can do is to always try to work as hard as you can

handle at your current fitness level. This achieves maximum calorie burn from the workout, and a more intense aerobic workout will keep your metabolic rate higher longer even after your workout has ended.

3. Do not exceed 60 minutes of high intensity aerobics per workout.

4. If you are a beginner, start with three aerobics workouts per week, between 20 to 30 minutes per workout. If 20 minutes is too long, break it up into two, 10-minute sessions. Keep the intensity low at the beginning and bring it up slowly. If you are on a treadmill, you have two choices to increase the intensity. You can elevate the treadmill or you can go faster. Once you are consistently doing three 30-minute aerobic workouts per week, you can add a fourth workout. Depending on your goals, you should be doing between three and six aerobic workouts per week, 20 to 60 minutes each.

Attention: Always listen to your body. If your knees or other joints start bothering you, slow down. You might be going too fast for your current fitness level or be doing too much too soon. Don't be in a rush to do more. It is better to start slowly and avoid injuries than do too much, too soon and hurt yourself. Results will come soon enough. If you injure yourself, you will have to stop completely and wait until you recover before you start again, and that will really hold you back. Remember: slow and steady wins the race.

***

Key # 3—Proper Nutrition

This subject has confused many people. In this section, I will try to clarify and sift through all the misinformation that surrounds proper nutrition and weight loss. I will give you the facts that most if not all experts agree on and the theories that are backed by many experts. I will also give you some of my opinions based on everything I have learned about proper nutrition and weight loss in my 12 years in the weight loss business. Using all this information and common sense, I will explain to you the best way to eat and how to eat not only for maximum safe weight loss, but also for overall great health. Let's start with common sense. If you look at the weight of the average American, it has gone up significantly in the past 30 years and continues to go up at a rate of one to two pounds per year. I have read a lot about the so-called fat gene that scientists claim has something to do with weight gain in some people. Although I agree that genes make some people more susceptible to weight gain than others, I do not think our genes are the reason for the massive weight gains we are experiencing these days. We have had these genes for at least the past 100 years. Genes do not change overnight; they change over thousands of years. Therefore, you cannot tell me that our genes have changed so much that in the past 30 years they are causing this massive weight gain. The one thing that has changed is not our genes, but our habits. Think about it, today we eat a lot more processed foods than ever before; the portion sizes have gone from small, medium, and large to LARGE, EXTRA LARGE, AND SUPER SIZE. It seems to me that restaurants are competing over who can serve the largest portions.

Something else that has changed is our reason for eating. These days, food is not just used to nourish our bodies, but for entertainment or to make us feel better. Take these large portions, combine them with the fact that most of us were brought up by parents telling us we should eat all our food, so much so that it is imbedded deep in our subconscious minds, and what do you have? The most overweight nation in the world. But don't worry; a lot of European nations are right behind us, and catching up fast! As I have already mentioned, the sole purpose of eating used to be for the nourishment of the body. These days we eat to make us feel better. We eat when we are depressed; we eat for entertainment; we eat because we are bored; we eat because there is food in front of us; we eat to satisfy emotional hunger; we eat because we are programmed to eat (like when you go to the theater and you get popcorn although you just ate dinner). All these extra calories have to go somewhere. Therefore, besides changing what we eat and how much we eat, we should start questioning why we eat and when we eat. If it is for any reason other than nourishing the body, we should not be eating.

I am a Greek-American and I lived in Greece for about 12 years, until the age of 15. In 1987, my junior high school in Greece had approximately 350 students and only one or two were obese and maybe another two or three were slightly overweight. Now I go back to Greece and see more overweight kids and adults than ever before. What has changed? When I was young in Greece, ice cream was a treat and we had it once or twice per week, if that, and only in the summer. The same went for all the other junk foods such as cakes, potato chips, and sodas. We only had them occasionally as a treat. We ate home cooked meals most of the time. Nowadays I notice that kids and grownups eat very differently. They eat a lot more junk food than I ever did when I was younger. The same thing has happened here. At this point 40% of our kids are considered overweight, and the number is growing and it will keep growing unless we do something about it.

With our busy schedules, we eat at fast food restaurants a lot more and I know there are many children who only eat fast food because both parents work and they have no time to cook at home. Ask yourself how often you eat a home cooked meal (TV dinners and canned food do not count) and how often you eat out. In addition to the fact that our diet has changed for the worst in the past 30 years, as I mentioned before, our activity levels have also gone downhill. I know people that drive to the end of their driveway just to pick up their mail even on a sunny day. How many able people do you know that take the elevator to get to the first floor? How many people do you know drive around the parking lot to find a closer spot? Our kids nowadays are not as active as they used to be. They spend a lot of their time indoors playing computer games instead of being outside playing sports or doing something active. Combine this with the fact that our kids eat worse than most adults do, and it is no wonder 40% of our kids are overweight. In addition to the change in our eating and activity habits, our food supply has been contaminated by hormones, preservatives, chemicals, and whatever else is being fed to the animals and plants we consume. Do you still think our genes have changed, or is it our eating and activity habits? Yes, I agree that some people have genes that predispose them to gaining weight more easily than others, but those genes were always there and when our diet was much better and we were a lot more active, they had no effect on our weight. Some people are just lucky that they were born with a body that can handle junk food better then others, but just because you look good does not mean that you will not benefit from eating better. Many skinny people out there have had heart attacks and other health problems.

The main point I want to emphasize here is that I believe genetics have little to do with the sudden weight gain we have been experiencing in the past 30 years. The main reason is the fact that our eating and activity habits have changed dramatically in the past 30 years and our food source has been compromised with additives, preservatives, hormones, pesticides and who knows what else.

Before showing you the best way to eat to achieve a leaner and healthier body, let me give you some facts about quick-fix diets. The vast majority of people who lose weight on quick fix diets gain all the weight back, and in some cases even more, within one to two years. There are quite a few problems with quick-fix diets. Let me explain. First, you make such a dramatic change in your eating habits that it is almost impossible to sustain long term. Eventually you will go back to eating the way you used to and you will gain all the weight back. I have seen this many times, especially with the Atkins diet. Another problem with diets is that if you lose weight by dieting only, as much as 25% or more of the weight you lose will be muscle. You do not want this to happen, because as you lose muscle your metabolic rate will slow down and weight loss will slow down along with it, until it eventually stops. This partly explains why on most diets you may lose weight initially but stop losing after a while. A third problem with quick-fix diets is that they might not be healthy for the body in the long run. I could write an entire book on all the diets out there that don't work, but let's not waste your time with what does not work; let's talk about what does.

First, keep in mind that in order to lose weight and keep it off for life, you need four keys, and proper diet is only one of the four keys. I would like to start with an undisputed fact: temporary changes will only give you temporary results; permanent changes will give you permanent results. Quick-fix diets only give you temporary results because you only make temporary changes. Let's face it, your current dietary habits are partly to blame why you are in the shape you are right now and only a permanent change in those habits will allow you to get to where you want to be and stay there. The best way to make permanent changes in your dietary habits is to change the way you think of food, make a few changes at a time, and plan your meals a week ahead of time until the new meals become habits. Also, learn from your slip-ups instead of getting discouraged. Everybody has slip-ups, but as long as you learn from them you will have fewer and fewer over time until you don't have any, except on special occasions. It takes 21 days for new habits to start becoming part of your life, so really try to stay focused for the first 21 days. I promise it will get much easier after that.

So now that we know the best way to incorporate the new changes into our lives let us figure out what dietary changes we should make in order to lose weight and achieve a leaner and healthier body for life. Of course, as you know there are much controversy and conflicting opinions when it comes to proper nutrition. I would like to start with what the experts agree on. These are the facts nobody can argue with: everybody should cut down on all junk food (potato chips, candy, cakes, ice cream, etc.), and sodas and all sugar drinks should be cut down or eliminated. Cut down or eliminate the use of salt, and limit amounts of oils and butter. Although some oils are beneficial, like olive oil, flax seed oil, and fish oils, you only need small amounts of them.Too much of these oils can still make you fat. Your diet should be made up of mainly cooked and raw vegetables, raw fruits, legumes/beans, and some starchy vegetables and whole grain foods. Do not eat when you are under a lot of stress, because stress compromises digestion. Try to drink at least six to eight glasses of water per day, although you can get away with less water if you are eating a diet high in fruits and vegetables. Eat slowly and chew your food well before swallowing. This will aid digestion. Before you eat anything, always ask yourself, "Am I physically hungry or am I eating for any other reason?" The bottom line is that we need to simplify our diet by reducing our consumption of overly processed foods like junk food and foods that contain white flour and refined sugars, and start eating more high nutrient dense unprocessed foods such as vegetables and fruits. In most cases, the less processed the food we eat, the better it is for us. There is a lot of controversy as far as meat goes. In my opinion, we should definitely have some kind of animal product in our diet, although in small amounts. I consider fish, dairy products, and eggs to be the best choices, although having other meats and animal products like beef, chicken, and pork once per week or so is OK too. Overall, having some kind of animal product three to four times per week is ideal, but make sure you keep it lean or low fat. Animal products have micronutrients that vegetable products do not have, and if you are a strict vegetarian, you should supplement your diet with the micronutrients you do not get from vegetables. Don't get me wrong, having junk food occasionally won't kill you, but junk food should be a treat that you have occasionally, not the foundation of your diet. If you eat well 80% to 90% of the time, you will stay in good shape, so enjoy the occasional cake and don't feel guilty about it as long as you eat well the rest of the time. Here is a complete list of my dietary recommendations:

My Dietary Recommendations

Note: The Food and Drug Administration has not evaluated these dietary recommendations. These recommendations are based on my own research and what I know to be true and effective. There is a food list in the appendix of this book that could help you with your food choices.

Most Important

- Eat as much as you can of cooked and raw vegetables every day. Try to eat at least six to eight servings per day, of which two to three should be raw. Include spinach, string beans, broccoli, artichokes, asparagus, zucchini, kale, cabbage, bok choy, Brussels sprouts, Swiss chard, red beets and their greens, dandelion greens, celery, cauliflower, eggplant, peppers, mushrooms. Try to eat a lot of green vegetables. Some great choices for raw vegetables are lettuce, tomatoes, sweet peppers, cucumbers, carrots, snow peas, green beans.
- Eat at least one cup of beans or legumes every day: chickpeas, black-eyed peas, black beans, green peas, lima beans, pinto beans, lentils, red kidney beans, soybeans, cannelloni beans, pigeon peas, and white beans.
- Eat at least four fruits every day, but you can have more: Apples, apricots, bananas, all berries, clementines, figs, grapefruits, grapes, kiwi, mangoes, melons, nectarines, oranges, papayas, peaches, pears, pineapples, plums, star fruits, strawberries, tangerines.
- Eat three servings of whole grains per day. Try to eliminate all white flour and other refined grain products such as white bread, crackers, pretzels, etc. Whole grains include whole wheat, barley, buckwheat "kasha," millet, oats, quinoa, and brown rice.
- Do not have more than one or two starchy vegetables per day. If you are trying to lose weight faster, do not have them at all. Starchy vegetables include corn, sweet potatoes, potatoes, butternut squash,

acorn squash, winter squash, chestnuts, parsnips, rutabagas, turnips, water chestnuts, yams, pumpkins, and cooked carrots.

- Cut down or eliminate as much as possible all junk food and overly processed foods. To get a better idea of what I consider junk food and overly processed foods, go to the food list in the appendix and look at "Foods that should be avoided like the plague."

Important

- You can eat one ounce or less per day of nuts and seeds. Nuts and seeds are good when unprocessed and unsalted; raw is best. Best choices include almonds, cashews, walnuts, pecans, filberts, hickory nuts, macadamias, pignolis, pistachios, sesame seeds, sunflower seeds, pumpkins seeds, and flaxseeds.
- You can use all spices and herbs. Go very light on the salt if at all.
- Condiments should be avoided, because most of them have too much sugar and/or salt. A little mustard is OK, and a little ketchup is OK, too.
- No more than one to two dairy products per day. Try to make one of your dairy product choices a yogurt (organic plain is the best choice). If you like fruit, cut up some fresh fruits and add to the plain yogurt.) Dairy products include milk, yogurt, and all cheeses. Make sure you eat plenty of green vegetables to get your calcium.
- You can have lean fish once or twice per week.
- Eggs that come from free-range chickens that eat a natural feed are fine. Having this kind of eggs 4 to 5 times per week, I consider fine. If you are trying to build muscle, having one egg right after your weight training working is a good idea. It provides the body with the complete protein it needs right after the workout. But remember, more is not better.
- Do not have more than one to two serving per week of any kind of meat or poultry.
- No sodas or juices of any kind, including fresh squeezed juices. You can use a little juice for cooking. Of course, if you had to choose between real juice and a soda, the juice is better, but the whole fruit will always be better than the juice.
- No butters, margarine, or any hydrogenated fats of any kind.
- Light use of olive oil; flaxseed oil is OK.

- You can have one coffee or tea per day if you really need it.
- No added salt of any kind.
- No artificial sweeteners or added sugar.

Notes:
- As long as 80% to 90% of your diet consists of vegetables, fruits, legumes, you are on the right track. Animal products should not exceed 20% of your daily food intake.
- On special occasions like holidays, birthdays, etc. having junk food or drinks like cakes, chips, sodas, candy, etc. in moderation will not have any major effect on your health or weight so go ahead and enjoy them if you wish.

In addition to the weight loss benefits you will achieve by eating the way I suggest, you will also experience other benefits such as more energy throughout the day; being able to think more clearly; and overall improvement of health, but don't take my word for it. Eat this way for six weeks and you will see for yourself. After you see the benefits, you will not want to go back to the old ways.

Key # 4—CONSISTENCY

Consistency is the fourth and most important key, because you cannot achieve any results without it. You cannot do something occasionally and expect to get results. You have to do something consistently to get results. Without consistency everything you do is a waste, as far as results go. Not being consistent is like trying to get from point A to point B by taking one step forward and then one step back. You can do that all year long and you will not be any further forward than you were when you started. Unfortunately, this is how most people work out. They start an exercise program, they might do it for a month or two then they stop. They lose all the gains they have made, so then they start up, stop agan, and the whole cycle starts all over. The year goes by and they are exactly where they were a year ago, and in some cases in worse shape than they were a year ago. Unless you stay consistent with your workouts, the same will happen to you. The question is, why can't most people be consistent with their weight loss efforts? Why, if we know how great exercising is and what its benefits are, can't we sustain an exercise program long term? I have given this question much thought and done a lot of research to find an answer, and this is what I have come up with after 12 years in the fitness field.

Anthony Robbins, a renowned motivational speaker, says, "Everything we do in life we do for two reasons, 1) to gain pleasure and 2) to avoid pain. The drive to avoid pain is greater than the drive to gain pleasure."

Think about it—I don't know about you, but I know many people who hate their jobs. Why don't they quit? They don't quit for two reasons, 1) the fear that they could not find another job that pays enough to sustain their lifestyle, which would bring lots of pain, and 2) the money they get from that job buys them things that bring them pleasure. Well then, you might think, if exercising is so good for you and supposed to make you feel great, and feeling great is so pleasurable, why don't more people exercise regularly? I think it is because we have become a "NOW" society. We want everything now. We want results now, not later; but results don't come until later and most people can't wait.

Let's analyze this. When you first begin an exercise program, you place yourself outside your comfort zone because exercising is a strain on the body. When you are outside your comfort zone, you are, to a certain extent, experiencing a degree of pain. Many people make matters worse by exercising too much when they first start their exercise program because they think they will get results faster by doing more. What they are doing is getting themselves even farther away from their comfort zone, and they experience even greater pain. Even though most people begin their exercise program with their goals in mind and how great they will feel when they get there (the drive to get pleasure), once, they start their exercise routine they start focusing on the immediate discomfort ("pain") they are going through. They then forget about the pleasure they will get when they reach their goal, and instead think about the pain they are going through right now. As we are a "now" society the immediate discomfort of exercising is more real than the future pleasure they will get through exercising, and as the drive to avoid pain is greater than the drive to gain pleasure, they quit.

Here are some ways you can motivate yourself to do the right thing consistently, whether it is exercising, eating right, or whatever else you need to do to achieve the results you want:

If you are a beginner or have not worked out for a long time, start slowly and don't exercise too much too soon. The mistake many people make is that they want results quickly, because they are very excited and want to get to their new body as soon as they can. As a result, they figure that the more they do the faster they will get there, but what happens instead is that the more they do the faster they quit. They get so far outside their body's comfort zone that they burn themselves out before they even see any results. My suggestion to these people is that they should start slowly and over time, as they get used to the workouts, make the workouts more intense. This gives to their body a chance to adapt and expand their comfort zone, thus avoiding burn out. For the exercise programs that involve modifying the diet also, people should start with the exercising part first before they make any big changes in their diet, because if they try to start exercising and change their diet too dramatically, they will overwhelm themselves with too much change and give up. They should try to make one or two changes at a time and as they get used to the new changes, make additional ones. In Chapter 3, I will explain in detail how to start an exercise program and how to progress.

If you have tried to start an exercise program in the past, but were never able to stick to it long enough to see results, the most likely problem is that although you start with your fitness goals in mind, you lose focus. Instead of concentrating on the end result and how great you are going to feel, you focus on the immediate discomfort of exercising. Once you focus on the discomfort of exercising, you start looking for reasons why you cannot continue to exercise.   Here is an exercise that will help you stick with your weight loss efforts: Write down the results you are looking for, making sure they are realistic. Write down how you are going to feel about yourself, and how others are going to feel about you once you have achieved the results you want. Try to build a vivid picture in your head of having already achieved your goals; picture how great it feels; and really believe that you can achieve the results you want. Every morning and every night look at what you have written, and try to feel how great it will be once you get there. By doing this every day, you will be motivated to keep exercising and keep doing whatever else you need to do to achieve your goals.

This is a way to motivate yourself to get pleasure, but earlier we said that the motivation to avoid pain is greater than the motivation to get pleasure. As a result, this motivation system might not work for some people because they find exercising and watching their diet and whatever else they need to do to achieve the results they want too much of a "pain." For these people, the drive to avoid the pain of having to exercise is greater than the drive to get the pleasure they would get by achieving the results they want. For these people, I have another suggestion: do the same thing as above and set the note aside. On a different note, write down how are you going to look and feel in one year from now if you don't start exercising and watching your diet. How much weight will you have gained? Then write down how you are going to look and feel in 5 years from now. Think about all the diseases you can develop by not doing anything; think about all the pain you will feel when you look at yourself in the mirror. Think about how tired and unhealthy you are going to feel. Write down how much worse it will get 10—20 years from now. Look at some older people and the pain they are going through right now because they did not take care of themselves when they were younger. Talk to them about the pain they go though every day because of the diseases they have developed, such as heart disease, diabetes, hypertension, osteoporosis, and many more because they did not take care of themselves. Think about how you will feel when you are older, thinking, "If only I had taken better care of myself when I was younger, how much better I would be feeling right now." Remember also that by being in good shape you will have fewer medical bills over your lifetime. Studies have shown that people who exercise have overall fewer medical expenses than people who do not. By getting and staying in shape, as well as avoiding a lot of future pain, you get to save some money, too. Now, think about this, you can avoid all pain that most likely you will feel at one point or another in the future by going through some minor discomfort now.

The choice is yours, a little discomfort now or a lot of pain later. If the future benefits you will get from exercising and eating right today do not motivate you to take action today, then the thought of all the pain you are likely to go through in the future if you continue on your present course with no change should motivate you. Every time you don't feel motivated to exercise or to eat right, think of all of the above.

In Chapter 3, you will find two more mental exercises that will help stay motivated. One quick note here: exercising itself does become pleasurable after a while, but most people quit long before that point. It is also important to note that learning to eat correctly is a matter of habit. Yes, it will take some time to develop the good habits but once established, eating properly will be second nature. The goal of **Live Your Way Thin** is to get you to the point where exercising and eating right is part of your life and will not require any extra effort; therefore enabling you to sustain the results with ease.

How long you live is not as important as the quality of the life you live.

You have to look at what you are hoping to achieve as a huge puzzle. Every action you take to move closer to the result you want (example: the ten minute walk, not having the doughnut after dinner, doing a weight training session, having water instead of soda) is one piece of the puzzle. By itself, it is nothing. It looks unimportant but as you put more and more of these seemingly inconsequential pieces together, they start forming a picture. Sometimes you have to put quite a few pieces together before you start seeing the picture, but before you know it, these strange looking, unimportant pieces complete a beautiful picture. Every action you take towards the results you want, as unimportant as it might seem at the time, does make a difference. Remember, a long journey is made up of small steps. Every time you want to eat a piece of cake, have a soda or do anything that will sabotage your progress, ask yourself this question: "Do I really want to have this piece of cake, or do I want to lose weight?" The cake will give you

short- term pleasure that you will regret later. How great will you feel when you lose the weight that you are trying to lose? Which is more important? However, if you do decide to eat the cake, which by the way is OK occasionally, then enjoy it.

CHAPTER 3

Start Building Your New Body

Getting Started

Are you ready to take action? In this chapter, I will help you take the first steps on your way to a beautiful, lean, and healthy body. I have broken the program down into four simple steps. All you have to do is follow the steps and you cannot fail. Before you start, read and familiarize yourself with all four steps.

Step 1

Define your fitness goals. What are you trying to achieve through this program? What benefits will you reap from achieving your fitness goals? Write your answers down clearly. If the benefits don't motivate you enough, write the consequences of continuing on your present course without changing anything. Remember what we talked about in Chapter 2—consistency. Go back and reread it if you don't remember. To help you with this process I have created a Goal & Attitude Questionnaire (see appendix). After you have completed it, read it at least once per day, and keep it somewhere that you can see it every day.

Step 2

After you have defined your fitness goal, start doing the following two mental exercises.

Note: Sometimes the only thing stopping us from achieving our goals is our own subconscious mind. Because many of us have failed so many times at losing weight, we have accepted the idea that we are always going to be overweight and that our body was meant to be this way. We start believing that we cannot achieve the body we want. Once you believe that you cannot lose weight, your subconscious mind makes sure you are right. I'm sure you have heard the saying, "Whether you think you can or you think you can't, you are right."

As I have already mentioned earlier in the book, the human body was meant to look fit, not overweight and unhealthy. All you have to do is remove the obstacles that get in your body's way and truly believe you will lose weight. When you truly believe you can lose weight, your subconscious mind, once again, will make sure you are right.

Below are two exercises you can do in order to reprogram your subconscious mind to help you achieve the body that nature intended you to have in the first place.

Exercise 1 (Do this exercise for 21 days straight.)

Sit or lie in a comfortable position, somewhere that you know you will not be disturbed. For 10—15 minutes see yourself with the body you want. See yourself being a person that loves healthy foods like fruits, vegetables, and legumes, and hates junk foods. Visualize yourself enjoying exercising and taking long walks whenever you can. See yourself in the present tense: make the picture vivid and smell, feel, see, and hear everything that is going on around you. Use all your senses to make the image as real as possible. Make the food that you try to give up taste bad, full of worms and other disgusting things. See yourself perform the activities that you need to do, such as aerobics and weight training, effortlessly and with pleasure. See yourself going through the workout successfully and anticipating the next opportunity to work out. It is important that you see yourself performing all the activities flawlessly and with ease. At last, see yourself with the body you want. Do not criticize yourself whether you can do it or not, just visualize it as if it is real.

The problem with change is that everybody has a self-image that his or her subconscious mind tries to uphold. If the self-image in your head is of somebody that loves eating all the wrong foods and hates any type of physical activity, it will be very hard for you to stick to any new changes that go against your self-image. If you first change your self-image to someone that loves doing the activities necessary to achieve your fitness goal, change will be much easier. The purpose of this exercise is to change the image that you hold in your head about yourself. This exercise really works, but don't take my word for it. Try it yourself and you will see. Earl Nightingale said it best, "You become what you think about."

If you want more information on how to change your self-image, read The New Psycho-Cybernetics by Maxwell Maltz.

Exercise 2

For the next 21 days, write down the following statements every morning as soon as you wake up and every night before going to sleep. As you write each statement down really believe it; see yourself doing it and do not question where you can find the time or how you can do it.

1. I love vegetables and I eat at least eight servings per day.
2. I love fruits and I eat at least four servings per day.
3. I do some form of aerobics every day for 30 minutes or more.
4. I do at least two weight-training workouts every week.
5. I love being active and I eat healthy all the time.

Before any goal can be materialized, you have to truly believe it in your mind.

Step 3

Start the workout routine. Do the workout that follows two times per week, skipping at least one day in between. Don't forget to change the exercises for each body part every three to four weeks.

Here I have a routine that I usually recommend to people that are just getting started. It is a simple routine. The weight training part of it should not take you more than 20 minutes to complete. You can do the aerobic part right after the weight training or separately. For more details, see Chapter 4 *The Workout Routines.*

Sample Workout

Warm Up

5 minutes walking on the treadmill, slow pace.

Resistance Training

Dumbbell Press (Chest)

1 set of 10 to 12 reps
Bend over Rows (Back)
1 set of 10 to 12 reps
Shoulder side raises (Shoulders)
1 set of 10 to 12 reps
Seated bicep curls (Biceps)
1 set of 10 to 12 reps
Lying dumbbell triceps ext. (Triceps)
1 set of 10 to 12 reps
Dumbbell Squats (All muscles in the legs)
1 set of 10 to 12 reps
Superman (Lower back)
1 set of 12 reps
Crunches legs down (Abs)
1 set of as many reps as you can. If you can do more than 30, pick a harder ab exercise.

Note: Don't forget to stretch after each exercise. You can find all the exercises and stretches in Chapter 5 *The Exercises*.

Aerobic Training

Walk on the treadmill or outside. Go slowly initially and gradually increase to a fast-paced walk. Do this three times per week, between 20 to 30 minutes each time. Skip a day in between workouts. As you become more aerobically fit, increase the intensity of the aerobic workout. Here are some tips on how you can do that:

• Speed up your pace.
• If you are walking outside and you want to increase the intensity without increasing the impact on your knees too much, do a power walk.
• If you are on a treadmill, you can go faster or you can increase the elevation. (Do not hold on to the treadmill.)
• You will burn more calories doing a power walk than if you do a slow jog.
• If you are significantly overweight, try to stay with low impact aerobics.

- The bike, the stepper, and the elliptical are great low impact aerobics.

You can choose to do the sample workout or pick your own exercises. Stay with this workout for at least four weeks. After four weeks, you may increase the intensity of the workout. In Chapter 4, I explain how to do that.

Step 4

Wait at least two weeks after you have started your workout before you start Step 4. In step 4, you begin to work on your diet. Waiting for at least two weeks will give you a little time to start getting used to the workout before you challenge yourself with new changes. If you have not been consistent with your workout routine, don't start on Step 4 until you are. Ideally, I would not make too many dietary changes during the first few weeks. Give yourself a chance to get used to the workout before you really start working on your diet.

The following are suggestions on how to go about changing your diet, so you will eventually be eating the way you should be eating for maximum health and weight loss. **Note: Don't be in a rush to jump ahead. Never move to the next step on the diet unless you have been 100% consistent for at least one week on the current diet step that you are on, and only move to the next step on the diet if you feel comfortable with the changes you have already made. Each step was meant to build on the previous step, so never skip a step. By the time you reach the last step you should be eating very close to my diet recommendations. Some people might start seeing results right from the fist step on the diet; you can choose to stay at that step or you can go on. Go on and get as close to my recommendations as you can, which by the way, you do not have to eat exactly to get results. As you will notice, the steps concentrate more on the foods you should be eating and not on the foods you should not be eating. The idea is if you eat all the foods and the amounts I suggest, you will not have any room for any bad foods.**

Note: *If you are a highly motivated person and would like to jump-start your weight loss, go to Chapter 6, "Jump Start your Weight Loss," and follow my dietary advice from that chapter for one month if you can. You may do it for a shorter time if you prefer. After that, follow the dietary advice below.*

Step 4a
a.   Eat at least one raw vegetable per day.
b.   Eat at least two cooked vegetables per day.
c.   Eat at least two raw fruits per day.

Step 4b
a.   Eat at least two raw vegetables per day.
b.   Eat at least two cooked vegetables per day.
c.   Eat at least three raw fruits per day.
d.   Eat at least two servings of beans per week.
e.   Eat one whole grain food, or unprocessed starchy vegetable per day.

Step 4c
a.   Eat at least two raw vegetables per day.
b.   Eat at least three cooked vegetables per day.
c.   Eat at least four raw fruits per day.
d.   Eat at least three servings of beans per week.
e.   Eat one whole grain food, or unprocessed starchy vegetable per day.
f.   Eat seafood at least once per week.
g.   If you eat junk food (see Food Chart in the Appendix), cut it down to no more than five servings per week.

Step 4d
a.   Eat at least three raw vegetables per day.
b.   Eat at least three cooked vegetables per day.
c.   Eat at least four raw fruits per day.
d.   Eat at least six servings of beans per week
e.   Eat two whole grain foods or unprocessed starchy vegetables per day
f.   Eat seafood at least two times per week.
g.   If you eat junk food, cut it down to no more than four servings per week.

Step 4e

a. Eat at least seven servings of vegetables per day, three of which have to be raw.
b. Eat at least four raw fruits per day.
c. Eat at least one serving of beans per day
d. Eat two servings of whole grain foods or unprocessed starchy vegetables per day.
e. Eat seafood at least two times per week.
f. If you eat meat or poultry, cut it down to no more than three times per week
g. If you eat junk food, cut it down to no more than two servings per week
h. Have one formatted food per day such as organic yogurt (has to be organic).

Step 4f

a. Eat at least eight servings of vegetables per day, three of which have to be raw.
b. Eat at least four raw fruits per day.
c. Eat at least one serving of beans per day.
d. Eat three servings of whole grain foods or unprocessed starchy vegetables per day.
e. Eat seafood at least two times per week.
f. If you eat meat or poultry, cut it down to no more than two times per week.
g. If you eat junk food, cut it down to no more than two servings per week.
h. Have one formatted food per day like organic yogurt (has to be organic).

Of course, in each step you will be having other foods too besides the ones mentioned. Just make sure by the end of the day you have eaten the food mentioned in the step. In the steps, I have included the food that will make the biggest impact to your weight and health; however, you should look at my diet recommendations below to see what other foods also you should consider adding to your diet. Make a copy of Step 4 and put it on your refrigerator or somewhere you can see it all the time and mark which step you are working on at the time.

My Diet Recommendations

Note: The Food and Drug Administration has not evaluated these dietary recommendations. These are my recommendations based on my own research and what I know to be true and effective.

Most Important
- Eat as much as you can of cooked and raw vegetables every day. Try to eat at least six to eight servings per day, of which two to three should be raw. Include spinach, string beans, broccoli, artichokes, asparagus, zucchini, kale, cabbage, bok choy, Brussels sprouts, Swiss chard, red beets and their greens, dandelion greens, celery, cauliflower, eggplant, peppers, mushrooms. Try to eat a lot of green vegetables. Some great choices for raw vegetables are: lettuce, tomatoes, sweet peppers, cucumbers, carrots, snow peas, green beans.
- Eat at least one cup of beans or legumes every day: chickpeas, black-eyed peas, black beans, green peas, lima beans, pinto beans, lentils, red kidney beans, soybeans, cannelloni beans, pigeon peas, and white beans.
- Eat at least four fruits every day, but you can have more: apples, apricots, bananas, all berries, clementines, figs, grapefruits, grapes, kiwi, mangoes, melons, nectarines, oranges, papayas, peaches, pears, pineapples, plums, star fruits, strawberries, tangerines.
- Eat three servings of whole grains per day. Try to eliminate all white flour and other refined grain products, such as white bread, crackers, pretzels, etc. Whole grains include whole wheat, barley, buckwheat "kasha," millet, oats, quinoa, and brown rice.
- Do not have more than one or two starchy vegetables per day. If you are trying to lose weight faster, do not have them at all. Starchy vegetables include corn, sweet potatoes, potatoes, butternut squash, acorn squash, winter squash, chestnuts, parsnips, rutabagas, turnips, water chestnuts, yams, pumpkins, and cooked carrots.
- Cut down or eliminate as much as possible all junk food and overly processed foods. To get a better idea of what I consider junk food and overly processed foods, go to the food list and look at "Foods that should be avoided like the plague."

Important
- You can eat one ounce or less per day of nuts and seeds. Nuts and seed are good when unprocessed and unsalted; raw is best. Best choices include almonds, cashews, walnuts, pecans, filberts, hickory nuts, macadamias, pignolis, pistachios, sesame seeds, sunflower seeds, pumpkins seeds, and flaxseeds.
- You can use all spices and herbs. Go very light on the salt if at all.
- Condiments should be avoided, because most of them have too much sugar and/or salt. A little mustard is OK and a little ketchup is OK, too.
- No more than one to two dairy products per day. Try to make one of your dairy product choices a yogurt; organic plain is the best choice. If you like fruit, cut up some fresh fruit, and add to the plain yogurt. Dairy products include (milk, yogurt, and all cheeses). Make sure you eat plenty of green vegetables to get your calcium.
- You can have lean fish once or twice per week.
- Eggs that come from free-range chickens that eat a natural feed are fine. Having this kind of eggs four to five per week, I consider fine. If you are trying to build muscle, having one egg right after your weight training working is a good Idea. It provides the body with the complete protein it needs right after the workout. But remember, more is not better.
- Do not have more than one to two servings per week of any kind of meat or poultry.
- No sodas or juices of any kind, including fresh squeezed juices. You can use a little juice for cooking. Of course, if you had to choose between real juice and a soda, the juice is better; but the whole fruit will always be better than the juice.
- No butters, margarine, or any hydrogenated fats of any kind.
- Light use of olive oil and flaxseed oil is OK.
- You can have one coffee or tea per day if you really need it.
- No added salt of any kind.
- No artificial sweeteners or added sugar.

Notes:
- As long as 80% to 90% of your diet consists of vegetables, fruits,

legumes, you are on the right track. Animal products should not exceed 20% of your daily food intake.

- On special occasions like holidays, birthdays, etc. having junk food or drinks, like cakes, chips, sodas, candy, etc. in moderation will not have any major effect on your health or weight, so go ahead and enjoy them if you wish.

CHAPTER 4

The Workouts

The Workout Routine

Unlike many workouts that are based on gimmicks and the latest Hollywood fads, all of the routines I show you here are based on scientific facts and theories. They might seem very simple to some of you, but working out does not have to be complicated. The simpler the workout, the more likely you are to be consistent, and remember: consistency is what gets results. Keep in mind what I said earlier about single sets as opposed to multiple sets; there is no difference in strength or muscle gain in the first four months of a workout if you are a beginner. However, there is another benefit to keeping your workouts short and simple even beyond four months. Let me ask you a question: what would be easier to fit into your day, a 60-minute weight training routine, or a 20 to 30 minute weight training routine? Which workout are you more likely to miss, the 60-minute one or the 20 to 30-minute one?

Here is some more good news about a shorter weight training routine: you can do a 20 to 30-minute weight training routine that could get you not just the same results as a longer weight training routine, but much better results. The keys to getting the most out of your weight training routine are the following: most importantly the form, the number of reps you are doing, the amount of weight you are using, and extremely importantly, the speed at which you are performing the reps. I will show you how to do all that next. The workout I will be showing you is nothing new. The credit for the development of this type of workout, which by the way is referred to as "high-intensity strength training," goes to Arthur Jones. Arthur Jones developed and introduced Nautilus machines in the 1970s. Another person that should get credit is

Wayne Westcott, Ph.D. He conducted a lot of research studies on high-intensity resistance training that proved the effectiveness of this type of training. Dr. Westcott is considered the foremost expert on strength training. I owe a lot of my own knowledge and expertise on the subject of strength training to his teachings and research studies. I would also like to add here that my clients at Olympus Personal Training & Weight Management, and myself, train this way and the results are great.

One of my clients is a perfect example of how a shorter weight training routine can be more effective than a longer one. Wendy used to work out with another trainer before she came to me. With the other trainer, she used to do 60 minutes of very intense weight training. It was so intense that the next day she would always be very sore and sometimes even the day after that. Because the workouts were so intense and long, she began dreading them and she would use any excuse to cancel. Nevertheless, she stayed with the trainer for over one year until she quit completely. When she came to me, it took me a while to convince her that all she needed was only 20 to 30 minutes of weight training done right, two to three times per week, unless she was planning to do bodybuilding. She agreed to try my way. Within one year of starting my simple 20 to 30-minute routine, she had achieved better results strength wise than she did doing the 60-minute routine of very intense training. The main difference for her results was not just because the routine was more effective, but also the fact that with my routine she was a lot more consistent. She actually enjoyed the workouts and she felt great after she was done, not in pain. She associated good feelings with the shorter routine and she did not dread it.

The bottom line here is that by keeping the workout routine short, besides being as effective as a longer workout if not more effective, the chances are you will be more consistent with it, and as I said, consistency wins the game.

IMPORTANT: If you are new to strength training, you cannot just start with high-intensity training. You need to give your body some time to adapt to strength training before you can push it. In the first few weeks of strength training, you should be concentrating on form and not on how much weight you are lifting. Once you feel comfortable with your form, then you can start pushing the weights. You want to make sure you are using a weight that is heavy enough to allow you to do between 8 to 12 reps per set.

Below I will explain how to put together a beginner's workout program. I will also explain how to put together a beginner's weight training routine and a high-intensity weight training routine. In the Workout Modification section of this chapter, I will explain how to modify the beginner's workout routine to help you achieve your personal fitness goals. Keep in mind you must do the beginners workout routine for at least four weeks before modifying it, no matter what your fitness goals. Keep in mind no matter what your reasons for working out are, your goal for the first month is to establish good exercise habits.

Terminology and General Rules

Terminology
Repetitions are referred to as reps
Sets consist of reps.

General rules for beginner's resistance training:
1. Change the exercise for each body part after two weeks.
2. If you are just trying to tone up your muscles you only need to do one exercise per body part, and for each exercise, you only need to do one set of 10 to 12 reps. Remember: more weight training will not tone the muscle any more. In most cases, the layer of fat that lies over the muscle prevents you from looking toned, and more weight training will not help you lose the layer of fat any faster. Remember the four keys.
3. If you do not mind gaining a little muscle and strength, after the first four to six weeks move to the high-intensity strength training. If you are a woman, do not worry about bulking up with the high-intensity strength training. Most women will not bulk up like a man even if they do the same workout. Doing the high-intensity workout will help you get stronger and really tone your muscles.
4. Until you feel you have correct form, keep the weights (or whatever form of resistance you are using) light.
5. When you perform your resistance training exercises, use resistance that is very challenging during the last one or two reps of each set (except in the first one or two weeks when you keep it light.)
6. Always warm up for 5 to 10 minutes by doing some light aerobic

activity, before doing resistance training, unless it follows your aerobic workout.

Putting a Beginner's Workout Together

Each exercise routine should consist of three parts: resistance training, stretching, and aerobic training. You do not need to do the aerobics at the same time you do the resistance training.

INSTRUCTIONS

Beginner's resistance training.

For the resistance part of the workout, I will tell you which muscle group to work and in what order. Stretching should be done with the resistance training. All the stretches are listed in Chapter 5. After each lift you perform, you should stretch the muscle group you have just worked. For example, if you have just worked your biceps you should do a stretch for the biceps immediately after you finish the set. I have grouped the exercises by the main muscle group they work. In Chapter 5, I have included couple of exercises and instructions on how to do them for each body part. For more exercises, you can go to www.StavrosM.com. and subscribe to my newsletter. I leave it up to you to choose which exercise you want to do for each muscle group. Make sure you change the exercise after two weeks. For example, if you are told to do one chest exercise for a set of 10 to 12 reps, this is what you have to do step by step:

1. Go to the exercise list and pick one exercise for the chest, using whatever type of resistance you prefer.
2. If this is the first time you have done this exercise, keep the weights light until you feel comfortable performing the exercise. Once you feel you have the form right, increase the weight so the last one or two reps you do are hard.
3. At the end of the set, do the stretch for the chest. The stretch for the chest will be listed in Chapter 5 under "Stretches."
4. Pick a new chest exercise every two weeks or so.
5. Repeat the process for each muscle group, until you have exercised all the body parts listed in your workout.

6.   If you would like a workout chart to help you keep track of the resistance-training exercises you are doing, the number of reps and sets you are doing for each exercise and the amount of weight you use, I can email you the charts that I use at my facility at Olympus Personal Training & Weight Management. They work great. There is no charge, just email me at stavros@stavrosM.com and in the subject line put Workout Chart.

Aerobic training

In Chapter 5, you will find a list of aerobic exercises. I have marked which ones are considered high impact and which ones low impact. If you are a beginner start with low impact aerobics and slowly move to higher impact aerobics if you want. You do not have to move to higher impact aerobics. However, although you should start with low intensity aerobics when you first get started, as you become more fit, you should try to keep increasing the intensity of the workout. When you do aerobics, you should always try to work out at the maximum intensity you can handle at your current fitness level.

Note: If you are a beginner, I suggest following the beginner's workout below for the first three to four weeks and than modify it as you see fit.

Beginner's Workout

I recommended this workout for anyone, male or female, who has never done any kind of resistance training on a regular routine ever or within the past six months.

Warm Up

5 to 10 minutes of a light aerobic activity.

Resistance training

Choose one exercise for each muscle group from Chapter 5. Perform the exercise in the order the muscle groups are listed. Note: keep the resistance light until you feel the form is right, and then make sure you use resistance that is challenging on the last 1 to 3 reps. Don't forget to stretch each muscle group after each exercise.

Muscle Group

Chest: 1 set of 10 to 12 reps
Back: 1 set of 10 to 12 reps
Shoulders: 1 set of 10 to 12 reps
Biceps: 1 set of 10 to 12 reps
Triceps: 1 set of 10 to 12 reps
Leg exercise: 1 set of 10 to 12 reps
Lower back: 1 set of 12 reps
Abs: 1 set of as many as you can.*

*For this exercise, if you can do more then 30 reps comfortably, change the exercise to a harder one.

Perform the above workout two times per week, skipping at least one day in between workouts.

Aerobics

Choose one low impact aerobic activity. For information on aerobic exercises and what
are considered low and high impact, go to Chapter 5.

Activity

Pick a low impact aerobics exercise and start with a 20 to 30 minutes workout at a low intensity.

Perform the aerobic workout 3 times per week. You can choose to do the aerobic workout right after your resistance workout or by itself; it is up to you.

Sample Workout

Warm Up

5 minutes walking on the treadmill at a slow pace.

Resistance Training

Dumbbell Press (Chest)
1 set of 10 to 12 reps
Bend over Rows (Back)
1 set of 10 to 12 reps
Shoulder side raises (Shoulders)
1 set of 10 to 12 reps
Seated bicep curls (Biceps)
1 set of 10 to 12 reps
Lying dumbbell triceps ext. (Triceps)
1 set of 10 to 12 reps
Dumbbell Squats (All muscles in the legs)
1 set of 10 to 12 reps
Superman (Lower back)
1 set of 12 reps
Crunches legs down (Abs)
1 set of as many reps as you can. If you do more than 30, pick a harder ab exercise.

Note: Don't forget to stretch after each exercise.

Do this workout two times per week, skipping at least one day in between. Don't forget to change the exercises for each body part every three to four weeks.

Aerobic Training
Walk on the treadmill or outside. Go slowly initially and gradually work up to a fast pace.

Do this three times per week, between 20 to 30 minutes each time. Skip a day in between workouts. As you get aerobically fitter, increase the intensity of the aerobic workout.

Here are some tips on how you can do that:

- Speed up your pace.
- If you are walking outside and you want to increase the intensity without increasing the impact on your knees too much, do a power walk.
- If you are on a treadmill, you can go faster or you can increase the elevation (Do not hold on to the treadmill).
- You will burn more calories doing a power walk than if you do a slow jog.
- If you are significantly overweight, try to stay with low impact aerobics.
- The bike, the stepper and the elliptical are great low impact aerobics.

Note: You can choose to do the sample workout or pick your own exercises. Stay with this workout for at least four weeks before modifying it. When you are ready to move on to the next level, check out Modifications A through G and pick the one that best fits your goals.

<u>High-intensity strength training workout</u>

WARNING: Do not do high-intensity strength training until you have completed at least four weeks of the beginner's strength training workout. In addition, a partner is a good idea to assist you with the changing of the weights and spotting you.

High-intensity strength training has two phases. **Phase One** is the building phase and **Phase Two** is the recovery and maintenance phase. Phase One, the building phase, is six weeks long and Phase Two, the recovery and maintenance phase, should be at least four weeks long, but it can be longer if you like. If you have achieved the strength and muscle mass that you want and you don't really care about getting any stronger or building more muscle you can stay at the maintenance phase much longer and do the building phase only for one or two weeks. VERY IMPORTANT: When you first get started with the high-intensity strength training you want to do the maintenance phase first for a few weeks before you start with the building phase. This will prevent you from getting sore from the first workout. After that just follow the six weeks on Phase One and four weeks or so on Phase Two.

Phase One (Building)

Pick the same exercises as the beginner's weight training workout. This workout, due to its high intensity, requires more recovery time. That is why you should do it only two times per weeks, skipping two to three days in between workouts. I also suggest that during this phase you try to sleep 8 to 9 hours for proper recovery and try to have some form of lean protein right after your workout. It does not have to be a lot of protein; I find organic eggs or egg whites to be the best choice.

The Workout

Pick one exercise for each body part, just like you did for the beginner's weight training workout. You are only doing one set per exercise (see sample below). Don't forget, you still need to warm up for 5 minutes.

Sample Workout

Resistance Training

Dumbbell Press (Chest)
1 set of 8 to 10 reps
Bend over Rows (Back)
1 set of 8 to 10 reps
Shoulder side raises (Shoulders)
1 set of 8 to 10 reps
Seated bicep curls (Biceps)
1 set of 8 to 10 reps
Lying dumbbell triceps ext. (Triceps)
1 set of 8 to 10 reps
Dumbbell Squats (All muscles in the legs)
1 set of 8 to 10 reps
Superman (Lower back)
1 set of 12 reps
Crunches legs down (Abs)

1 set of as many reps as you can do super slow. If you do more than 20, pick a harder ab exercise.

The main difference between this workout and the beginner's workout is the speed at which you will be performing the reps and the fact you will be super setting all the exercises except the lower back and ab exercises.

How fast the reps should be done?

Each rep should be performed through the full rage of motion for the exercise, at a slow pace. Each rep should be six seconds long. You should take two seconds for the lifting phase of the exercise and four seconds for the lowering phase of the exercise. That is how you get to the six seconds for the whole rep. It is very important that you are very accurate with the speed of the movements. It helps to use a metronome to keep you on pace, or you can have your partner count out loud, one thousand one, one thousand two and so on.

How heavy should the weights be?

Use a weight for each exercise that allows you do perform 8 to 10 reps with good form, taking two seconds for the lifting phase and four seconds for the lowering phase. If you can do more than 10 reps with good form and at the right speed, make the weights heavier next time you do the same exercise. It is very important that you fail within 8 to 10 reps. (Fail means that you can no longer to the exercise with good form, and or at the right speed, six seconds for the whole rep.)

How do I super set?

In the initial set, once you can no longer lift the weight with good form and at the right speed (two seconds for the lifting phase and four seconds for the lowering phase), stop. Lower the weights by 10% to 20% and with no rest in between, do as many more reps at the correct speed as you can. Usually you should get another 2 to 4 reps out of it.

To make it easier and faster to drop weights, have the weights ready for the super set. If you are using a barbell, set the weights up so it is easy to remove 10% to 20% of the weight from the bar. It is very important that you take no rest at all between the two sets. You can rest between exercises.

Example:

Let's say you are doing the dumbbell press. You start with 20-pound dumbbells. When you are lifting the dumbbells it should take you two seconds and when you are lowering them it should take you four seconds. Let's say at the ninth rep you can no longer lift the dumbbells at the right speed (two seconds). You drop the dumbbells and grab the 15-pound dumbbells that you have set nearby, and you continue with two seconds lifting and four seconds lowering. Once you can no longer control the speed, stop. You will feel a burning sensation with this workout. Try to work through it the best you can. Keep in mind you only need to do one super set per exercise, so really focus on doing it right and slow.

How long should I wait between exercises.

You should wait anywhere from one to two minutes, depending on how much time you have available for your workout. The whole strength training routine should take between 20 to 30 minutes.

Phase Two (Recovery/Maintenance)

Phase Two is exactly like Phase One but without the super setting. In other words, once you can no longer perform the exercise at the right speed, you just stop without going into the second set, referred to as the super set. It is very important that you really concentrate when you are doing each set and make sure you push it to the max. You should feel a burning sensation during the end of the set. Try to push through it and only stop when you really cannot control the speed any longer. Keep in mind you are only doing one set per exercise, so try to do that set perfectly. It is OK to loosen up your form on the last one or two reps as long as the speed of the reps is maintained, but make sure you keep the exercise safe. As I said earlier, it is a good idea to have a partner to spot you with this type of training.

How often can I do this workout?

Because Phase Two is less intense, you can do this workout three times per week, skipping only one day between workouts. You can still do it two times per week, as in Phase One, if you choose to do so.

If you have any questions, please feel free to email me at Stavros@stavrosM.com . I try to answer all my email as soon as possible. In the near future, I will be coming up with a video demonstration on how to perform a high-intensity strength training workout. For more information, you can go to my web site, www.stavrosM.com .

Note: If you are a beginner, I suggest following the beginner's workout for the first three to four weeks and than modify it as you see fit. On how to modify your beginner's workout and when you should switch to the high-intensity strength training routine, go to Workout Modifications in this chapter.

Workout Modifications

Modification A (Female)

If your goal is to lose weight and tone up but you do not want to bulk up, and you don't care to get any stronger, this is how you should modify your beginner's workout:

1. You could add one more resistance-training workout per week, but is not necessary.
2. Stay with one exercise per muscle group and do only one set per exercise of 10 to 12 reps.
3. Make sure whatever resistance you chose is challenging. If it is not, then increase the resistance.
4. Keep increasing the intensity of the aerobic workouts as long as you can handle it, but if you are significantly overweight keep the impact low.
5. Increase the duration of the aerobic workouts up to 60 minutes, but not longer. You can still do some shorter workouts (30 minutes) if you want.
6. Increase the number of aerobic workouts up to six per week. Try not to do high impact aerobics back to back, and always take a full day's rest at least once per week.

7. If, after you have lost some weight, you realize that a muscle group or groups are underdeveloped, you can do two sets per exercise for that muscle group.

Modification B (Female)

If your goal is lose some weight, tone your body, and add some muscle and get stronger, this is how you should modify your beginner's workout:

1. Switch to the high-intensity strength training. Make sure you start with Phase Two for the first two weeks.
2. Alternate Phase One and Phase Two of the high-intensity strength training every six weeks.
3. Make sure whatever resistance you chose is challenging; if not, increase the resistance.
4. Keep changing the exercises for each muscle group every three to four weeks.
5. Keep increasing the intensity of the aerobic workouts as long as you can handle it.

6. Don't increase the duration of the aerobic workouts over 45 minutes.
7. Increase the number of aerobic workouts up to five times per week.

Modification C (Female)

If your goal is to tone up and to build some muscle, and weight loss is not a main concern, this is how you should modify your beginner's workout:

1. Switch to the high-intensity strength training workout. Make sure you start with Phase Two for the first two weeks.
2. Alternate between the phases as follows: six weeks on Phase One and four weeks on Phase Two.
3. If you have thin legs and you need to build them up a little, add the

following exercises. You can find instructions on these exercises at my web site, www.stavrosM.com.

a. Leg Curls (hamstrings)
b. Leg Extensions (quads)
c. Leg Adduction (adductors)

Note: If you have bulky legs, do not do the above exercises. These exercises are only for people that need to build their legs up.

4. Make sure whatever resistance you chose is challenging; if not, increase the resistance.
5. Keep increasing the intensity of the aerobic workout as long as you can handle it.
6. Don't increase the duration of the aerobic workouts over 30 minutes.
7. Do not do more then four aerobic workouts per week.

Modification D (Male)

If your goal is to lose weight, tone your muscles, and get in good overall shape, and you don't care to increase your muscle mass or your strength, this is how you should modify your beginner's workout. Note: Although this workout is not for bulking up or for increasing strength dramatically, you will still gain some muscle and you will get stronger over time, but not to the same degree as if you were doing a workout for building muscle mass or for building strength.

1. You can choose to add one more resistance training workout.
2. Stay with one exercise per muscle group and do only one set per exercise of 10 to 12 reps.
3. Make sure whatever resistance you chose is challenging; if not, increase the resistance.
4. Keep increasing the intensity of the aerobic workouts as long as you can handle it, but if you are significantly overweight keep the impact low.
5. Increase the duration of the aerobic workouts up to 60 minutes, but no longer. You can still do some shorter workouts of 30 minutes if you want.
6. Increase the number of aerobic workouts up to six per week. Try not

to do high impact aerobics back to back, and always take a full day's rest at least once per week.

7. If, after you have lost some weight, you realize that a muscle group or groups are underdeveloped, then you can do two sets per exercise for that muscle group.

Modification E (Male)

If your goal is to lose some weight and build some muscle, this is how you should modify your beginner's workout:

1. Switch to the high-intensity strength-training workout. Make sure you start with Phase Two for the first two weeks.
2. Alternate between the phases as follows: six weeks on Phase One and four weeks on Phase Two.
3. If you have thin legs and you need to build them up a little, add the following exercises. You can find instructions on these exercises at my web site, www.stavrosm.com.

   a. Leg Curls (Hamstrings)
   b. Leg Extensions (Quads)
   c. Leg Adduction (Adductors)

4. Make sure whatever resistance you chose is challenging; if not, increase the resistance.
5. Change the exercise you do for each muscle group every two weeks.
6. Keep increasing the intensity of the aerobic workouts as long as you can handle it.
7. You can increase the duration of the aerobic workouts up to 45 minutes.
8. Increase the number to aerobic workouts up to five per week.

Modification F (Male or Female)

If your goal is to build muscle and you have no weight to lose, then this is how you should modify your beginner's workout:

1. Switch to the high-intensity strength training workout. Make sure you start with Phase Two for the first two weeks.
2. Alternate between the phases as follows: six weeks on Phase One and four weeks on Phase Two.
3. If you have thin legs and you need to build them up a little add the following exercises. You can find instructions on these exercises at my web site, www.stavrosM.com.
   a. Leg Curls (Hamstrings)
   b. Leg Extensions (Quads)
   c. Leg Adduction (Adductors)

4. Make sure whatever resistance you chose is challenging; if not, increase the resistance.

5. Use weight instead of tubing for this goal; you will get a better workout.

6. Increase the weight for all the exercises to the point that sometimes you will not be able to do all 10 reps.

7. It is OK to cheat a little bit on the last one or two reps to complete the set, as long as you do not compromise safety.

8. Change the exercises you do for each muscle group every two weeks.

9. Do only three aerobic workouts per week, every other day, between 20 to 30 minutes each.

Important notes and advice

If you reach your goal, or your goal has changed, feel free to change the workout to suit your needs. Keep in mind that you will have weeks when you will be very busy and might not have enough time to do all your workouts. If that happens, just do the minimum, which is lifting once per week. If you resistance train once per week, that is enough to sustain the results that you achieved from your previous resistance training workouts. Two to three times a week is the ideal. The minimum for aerobic training to sustain your current aerobic fitness is three times per week for 20 minutes. Although three aerobic workouts per week of 20 minutes each is enough to sustain your current aerobic fitness, it might not be enough to sustain your current weight, because your weight is influenced by your diet, too. If your diet for that week was bad, you still might gain some weight. My suggestion to you is on those bad weeks when you do not have enough time to exercise as much as you would like, try to be extra careful with your eating habits.

CHAPTER 5

The Exercises

Resistance Training Exercises

<u>**Exercises that work the Chest:**</u>

Dumbbell Press

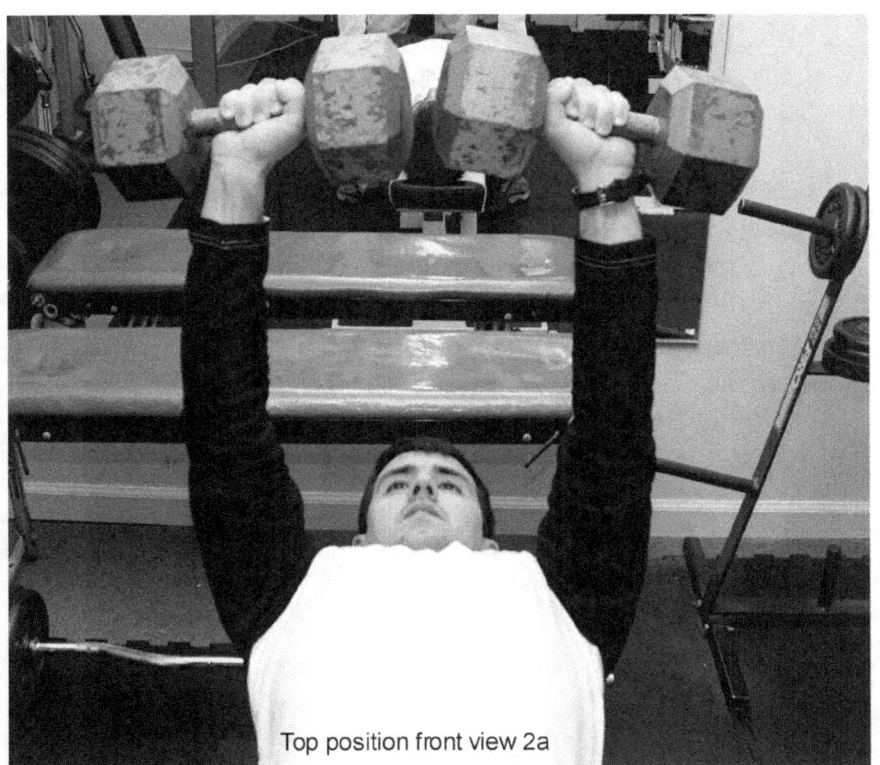

Top position front view 2a

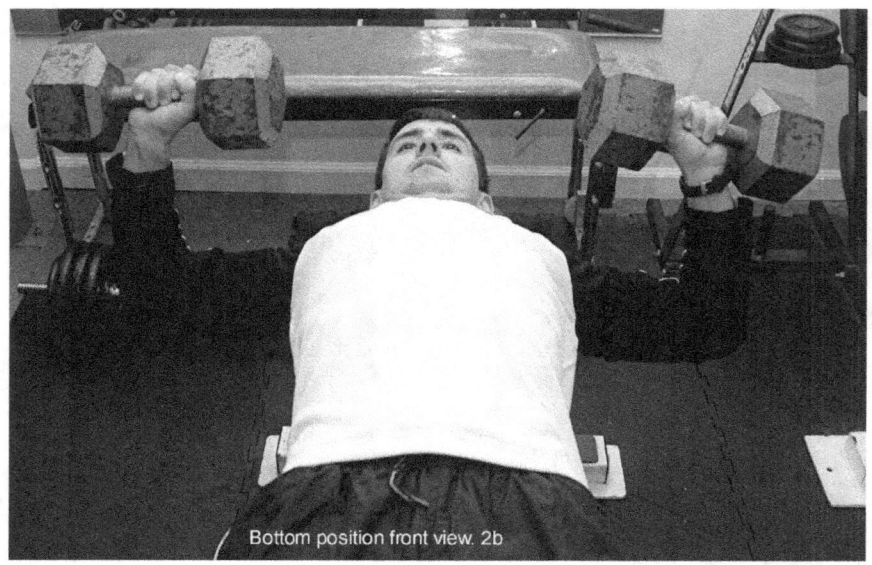

Bottom position front view. 2b

Main Muscle worked: Pectoralis major (chest)

Execution of the Exercise: Refer to pictures 2a, 2b

1. Start by lying down on the bench and getting the dumbbells directly over your chest. If you are not too tall, you can place your feet on the bench; but if you are tall enough and can place your feet on the floor without arching your back, that is fine.

2. Begin the exercise by bringing the elbows down nice and slowly, and as in the bench press make sure your elbows stay out to the sides. Your forearms should be pointing straight up at all times.

3. Once the elbows line up with your shoulders or slightly below, stop and bring the dumbbells up again to the starting position. Make sure your elbows stay out to the sides. You should be able to draw a straight line through the chest from one elbow to the other. Note: If your shoulders bother you in this position, bring your elbows in a little bit.

Chest press with tubing

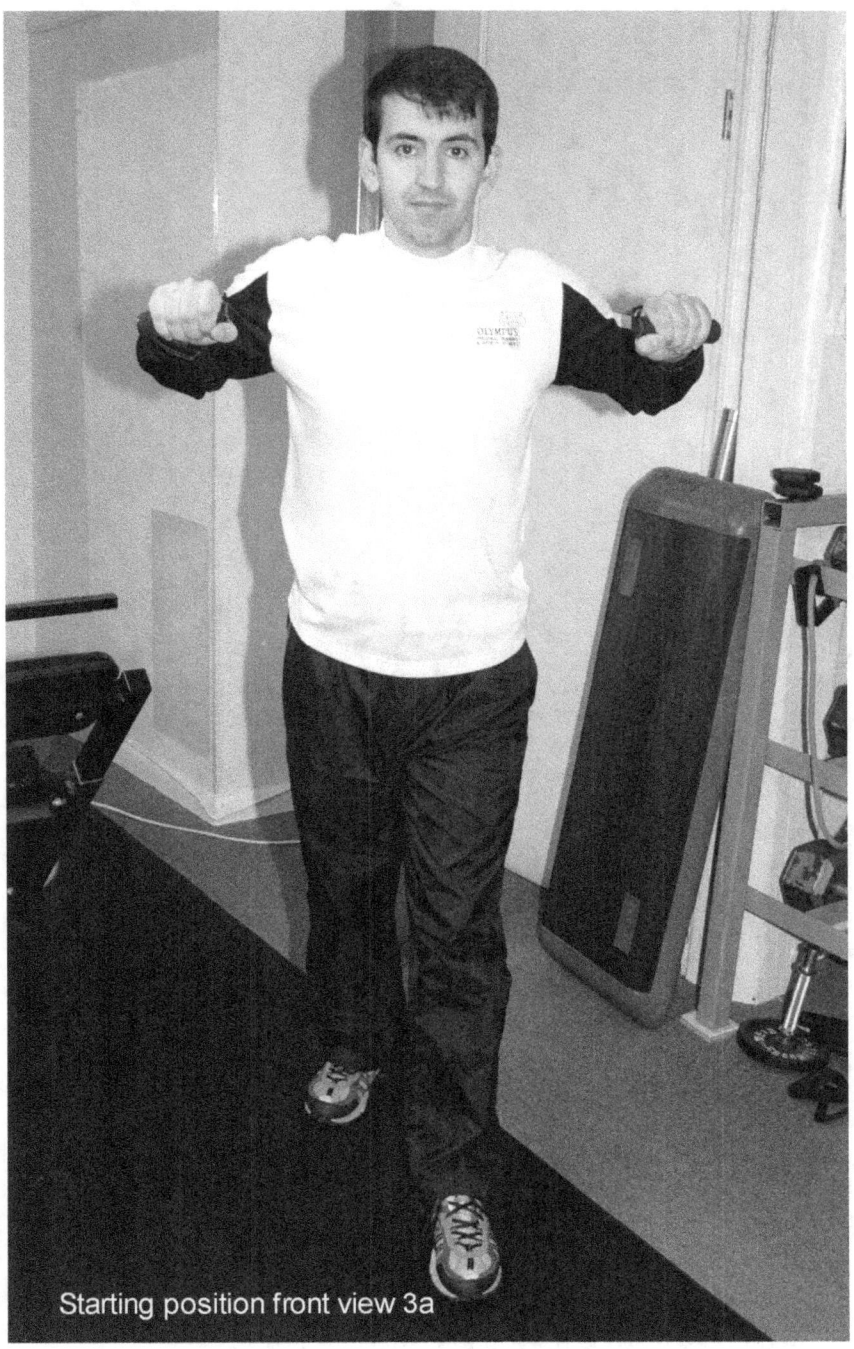

Starting position front view 3a

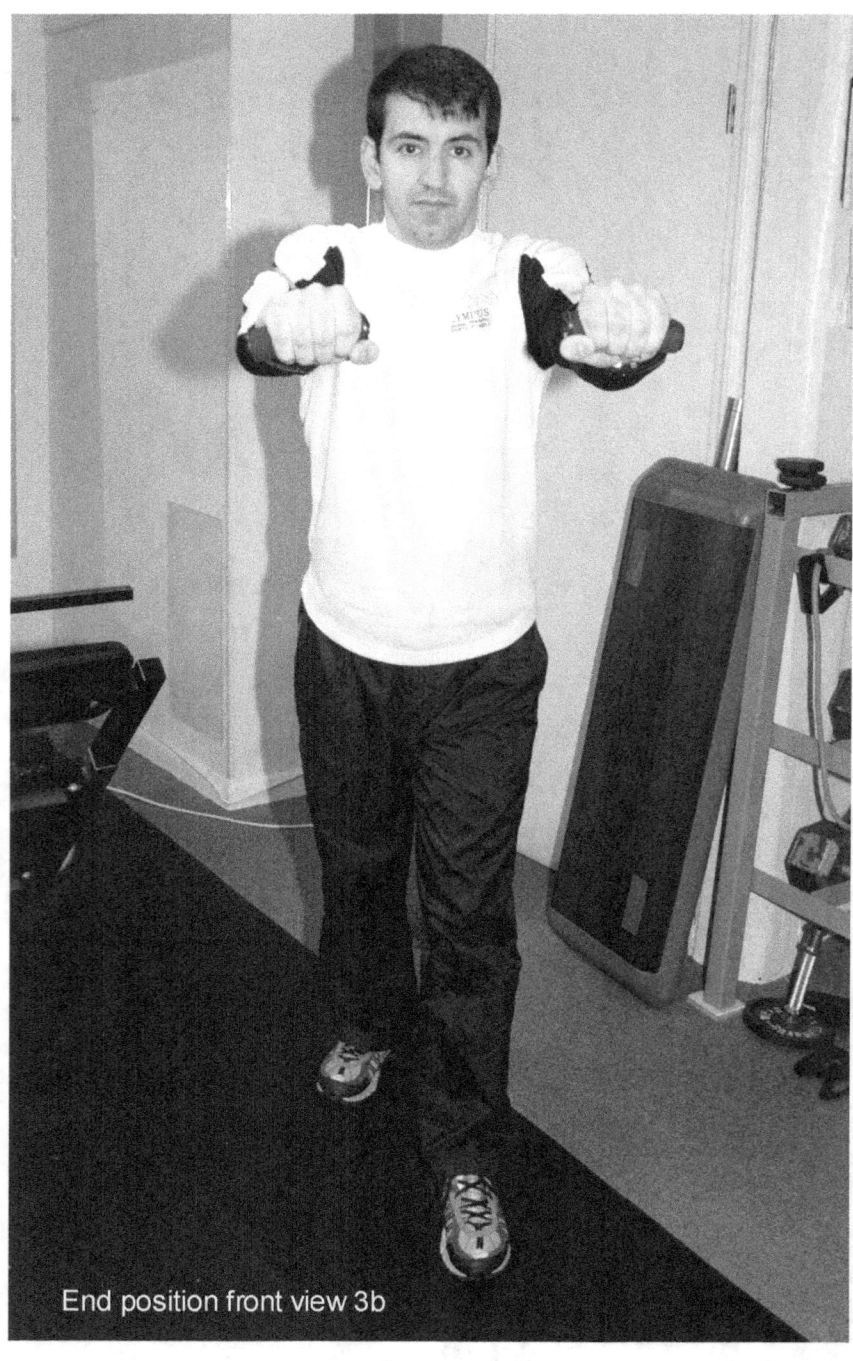

End position front view 3b

<u>Main Muscle worked</u>: Pectoralis major (chest)
<u>Execution of the Exercise</u>: Refer to pictures 3a, 3b

1. Get into position as in picture 3a. Keep your elbows high and your wrists straight. Your body should lean slightly forward and your feet should be one in front of the other.
2. Keeping your body leaning forward, extend your arms to a straight position (picture 3b).
3. Make sure you return your arms nice and slowly to the starting position.

Exercises that work the Back

Dumbbell Bent Over Row

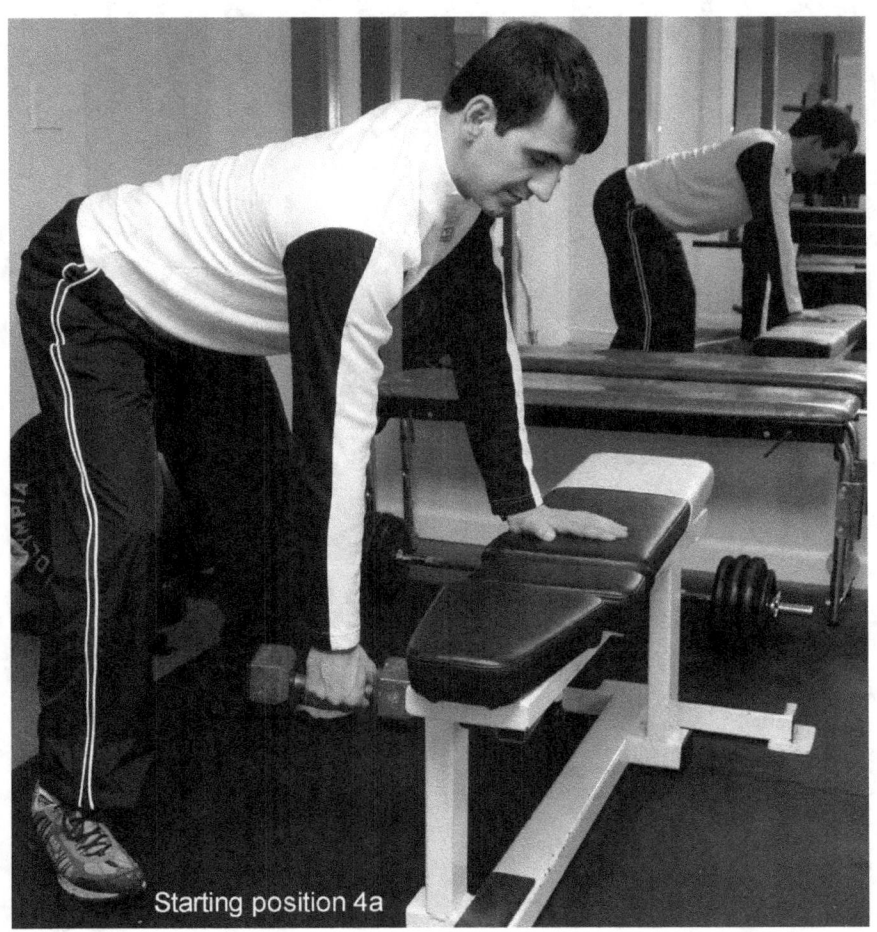

Starting position 4a

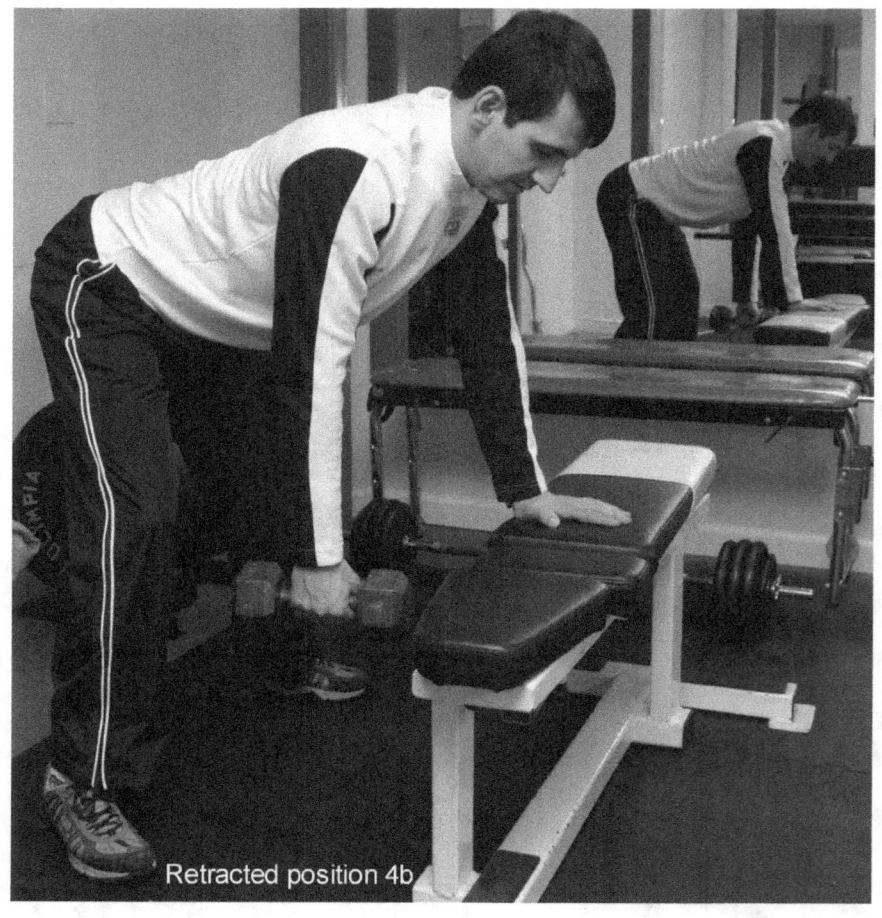

Retracted position 4b

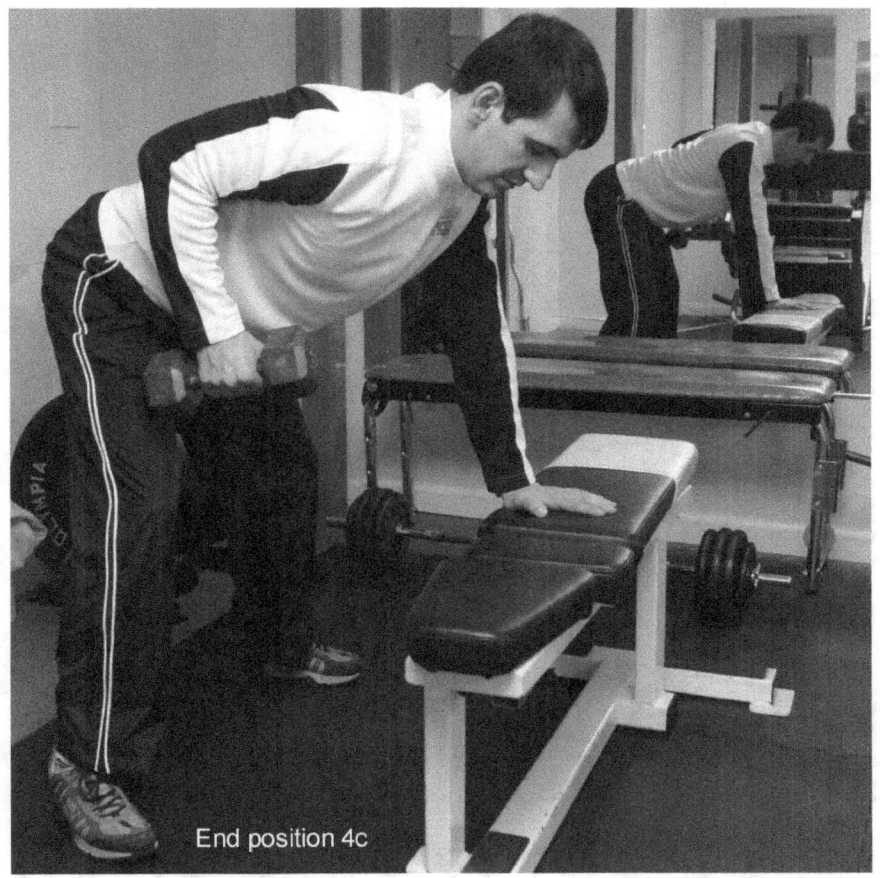

End position 4c

Main Muscles worked: Latissimus dorsi, Rhomboid major and minor, middle trapezius (back).

Execution of the Exercise: Refer to pictures 4a, 4b, 4c.

1. Start with your feet wide, back straight and parallel to the ground, buttocks sticking out at the back and knees slightly bent. Place a hand on a bench for support. With the other hand grab the dumbbell, keep your back straight, and let your shoulder drop down (picture 4a).

2. Begin the movement by first retracting your shoulder blade. At this point, your arm should be straight (picture 4b)

3. Once you have fully retracted the shoulder blade, bring the elbows up to the side as if you are doing a row. Stop when the elbow is at the same height as the back, then drop the arm and shoulder down and repeat the process. Make sure your back stays straight throughout

the exercise and your forearm is always pointing down to the ground (picture 4c).

Seated Row with tubing

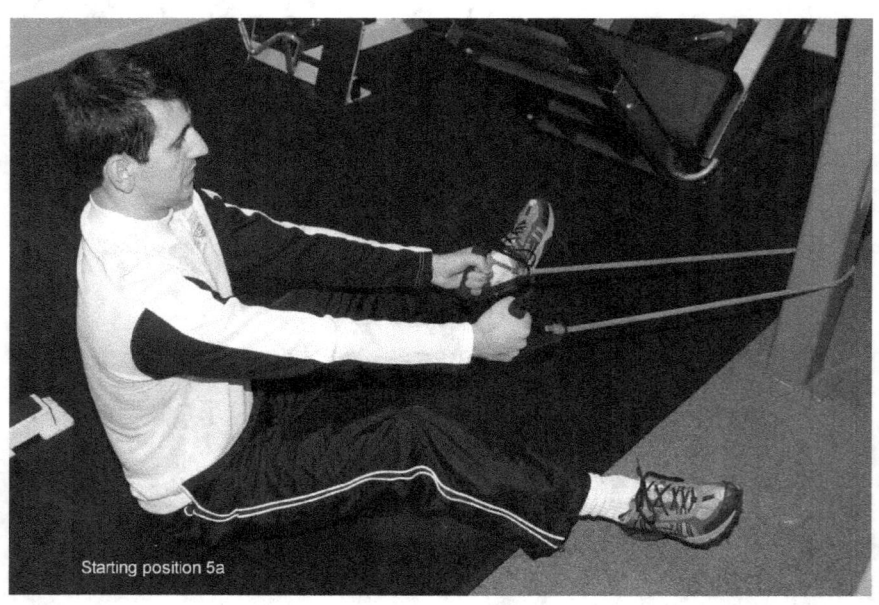

Starting position 5a

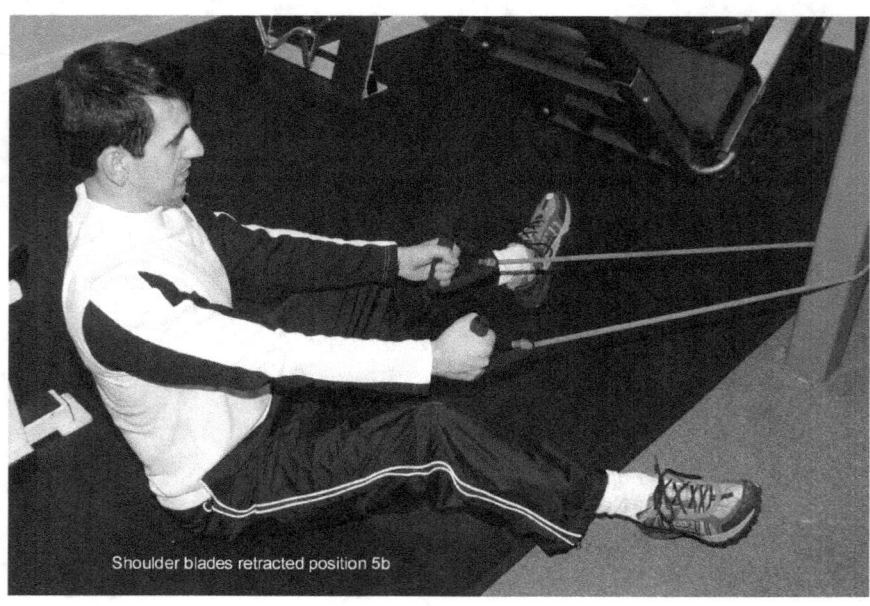

Shoulder blades retracted position 5b

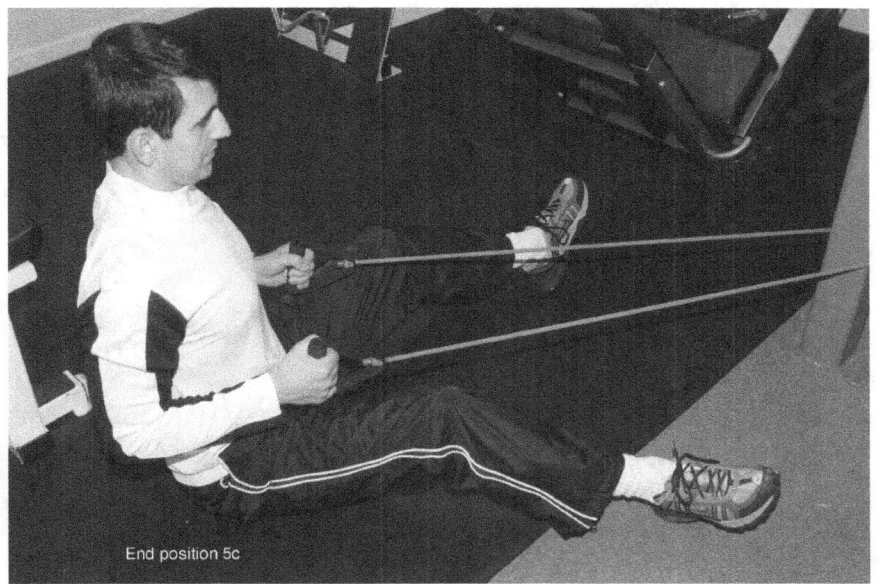

End position 5c

Main Muscles worked: Latissimus dorsi, rhomboid major and minor, middle trapezius (back).

Execution of the Exercise: Refer to pictures 5a, 5b, 5c.

1. Begin the exercise with your spine straight and your arms and shoulders pulled forward (picture 5a).

2. First, retract your shoulder blades, keeping your arms and body straight. (picture 5b).

3. Once your shoulder blades are fully retracted, pull the elbows back until they are lined up with your body or slightly behind you (picture 5c).

Exercise that work the Shoulders

Shoulder side raises

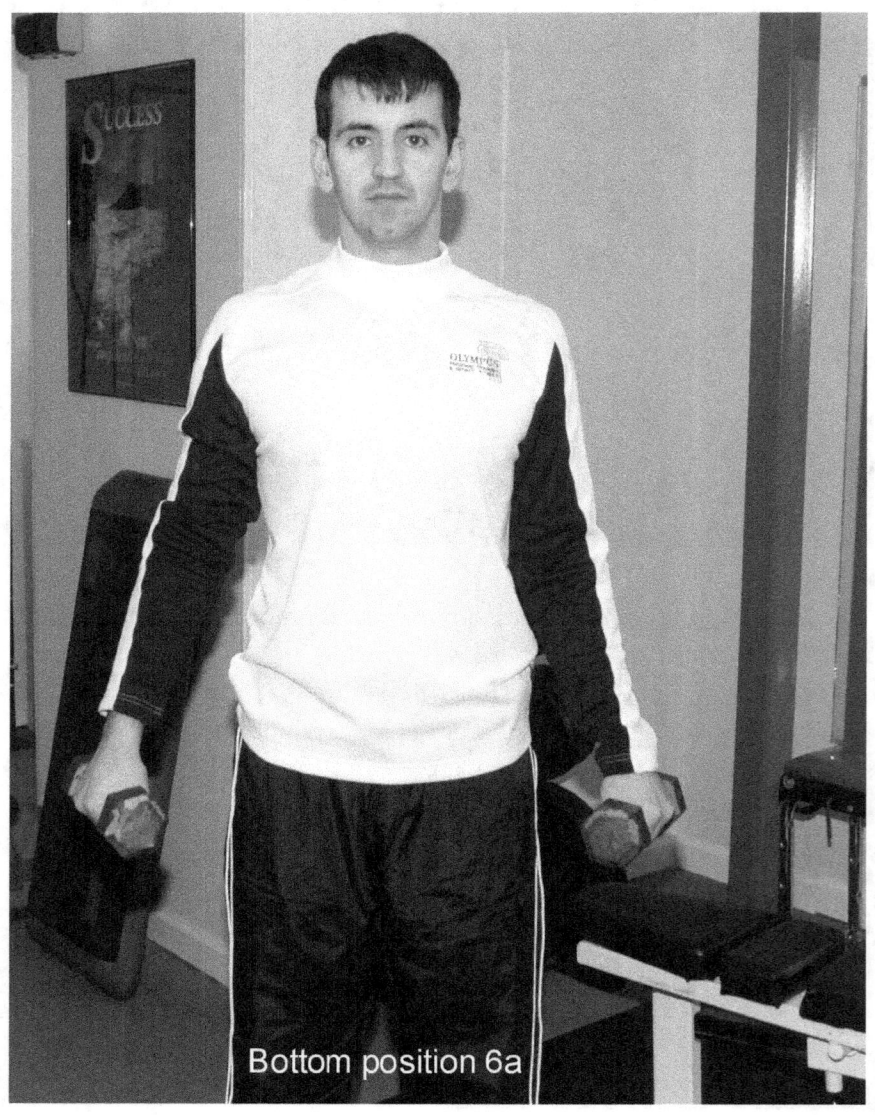

Bottom position 6a

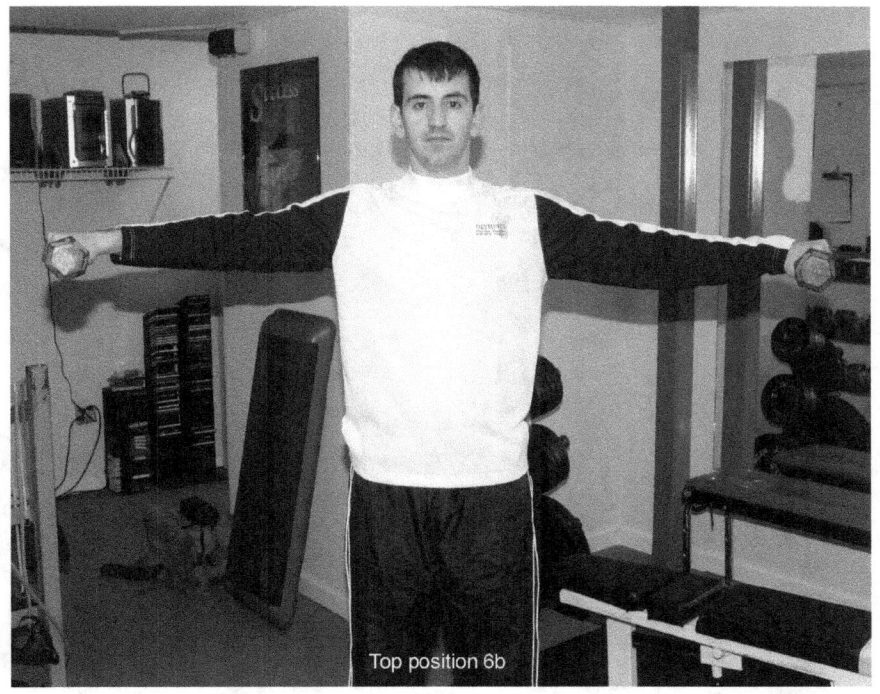

Top position 6b

Main Muscles worked: Deltoids (shoulder)

Execution of the Exercise: Refer to pictures 6a, 6b.

1. Keep your feet hip width apart, your elbows very slightly bent and your arms at your sides. The weights should not touch your sides (picture6a).

2. Begin by raising your elbows shoulder height or slightly below, keeping the angle of the elbow the same at all times. Do not concentrate on the dumbbells. Think of the elbows going up and down. The elbow should be frozen at a slight angle (picture 6a).

3. Pause for a brief second and then lower the elbows slowly until you reach the bottom position again.

Shoulder raises with tubing.

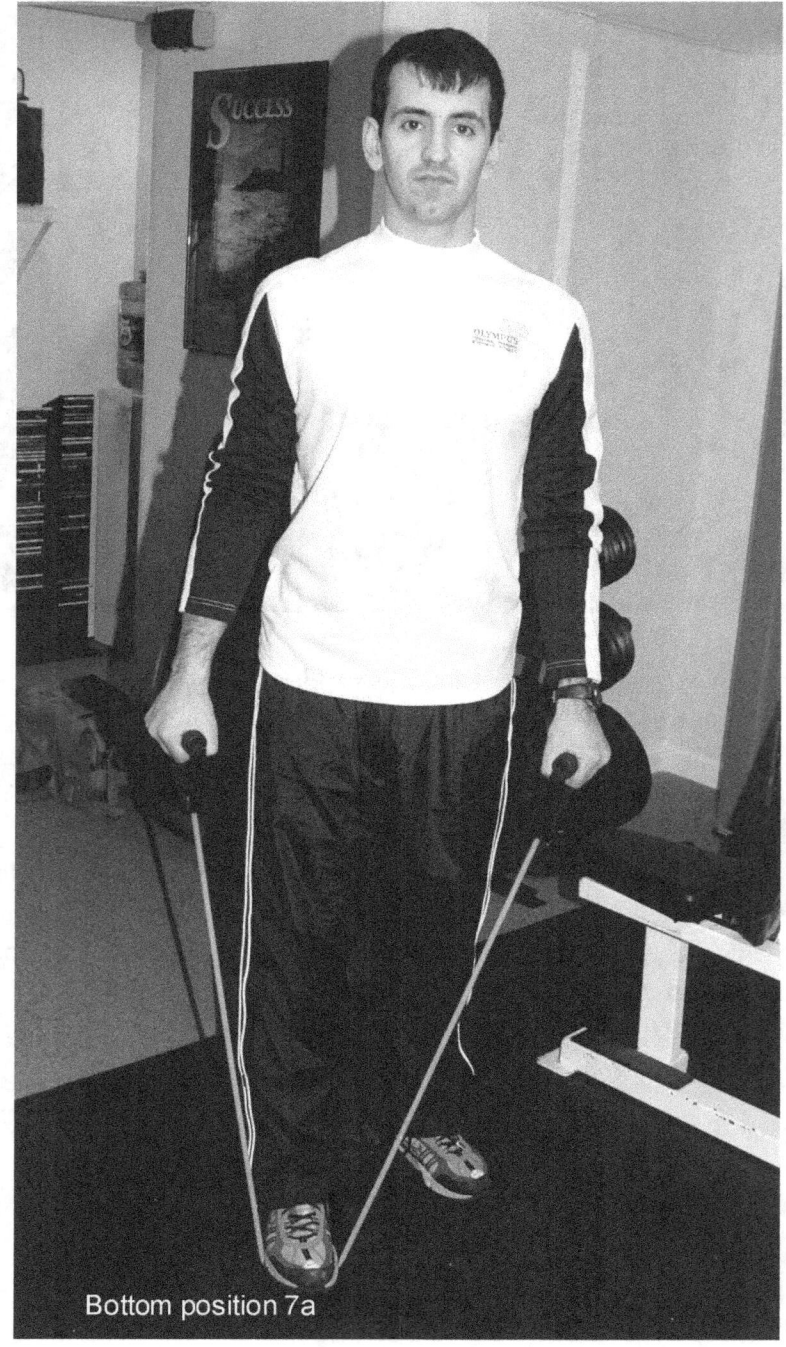

Bottom position 7a

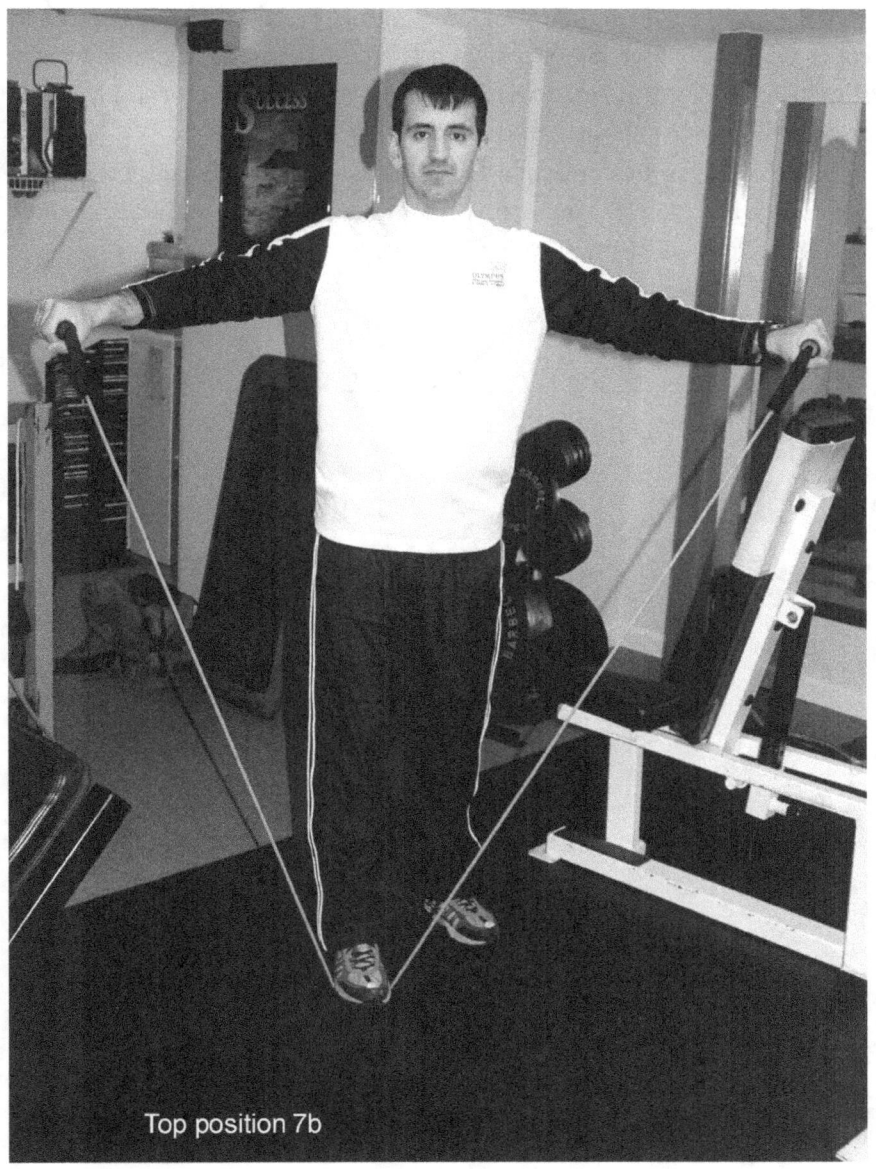

Top position 7b

Main Muscles worked: Deltoids (shoulder)
Execution of the Exercise: Refer to pictures 7a, 7b.

1. Begin by stepping on the middle of the tubing at the centerline of
    your body right in front of you. Your arms should be straight with
    a slight bend at the elbows and your palms should be facing in
    (picture 7a).

2. Think of bringing your arms up as a unit. Your arms should come up to shoulder height or slightly below, keeping the elbows at a slight angle. Keep in mind that your arms should not be completely to the side but rather slightly to the front (picture 7b).

3. Once you have reached the top, pause for a brief second and go down nice and slowly. Your arms should never come together, and there should be tension in the tubing at all times.

Exercises that work the Biceps (Front of Arms)

Seated dumbbell curls

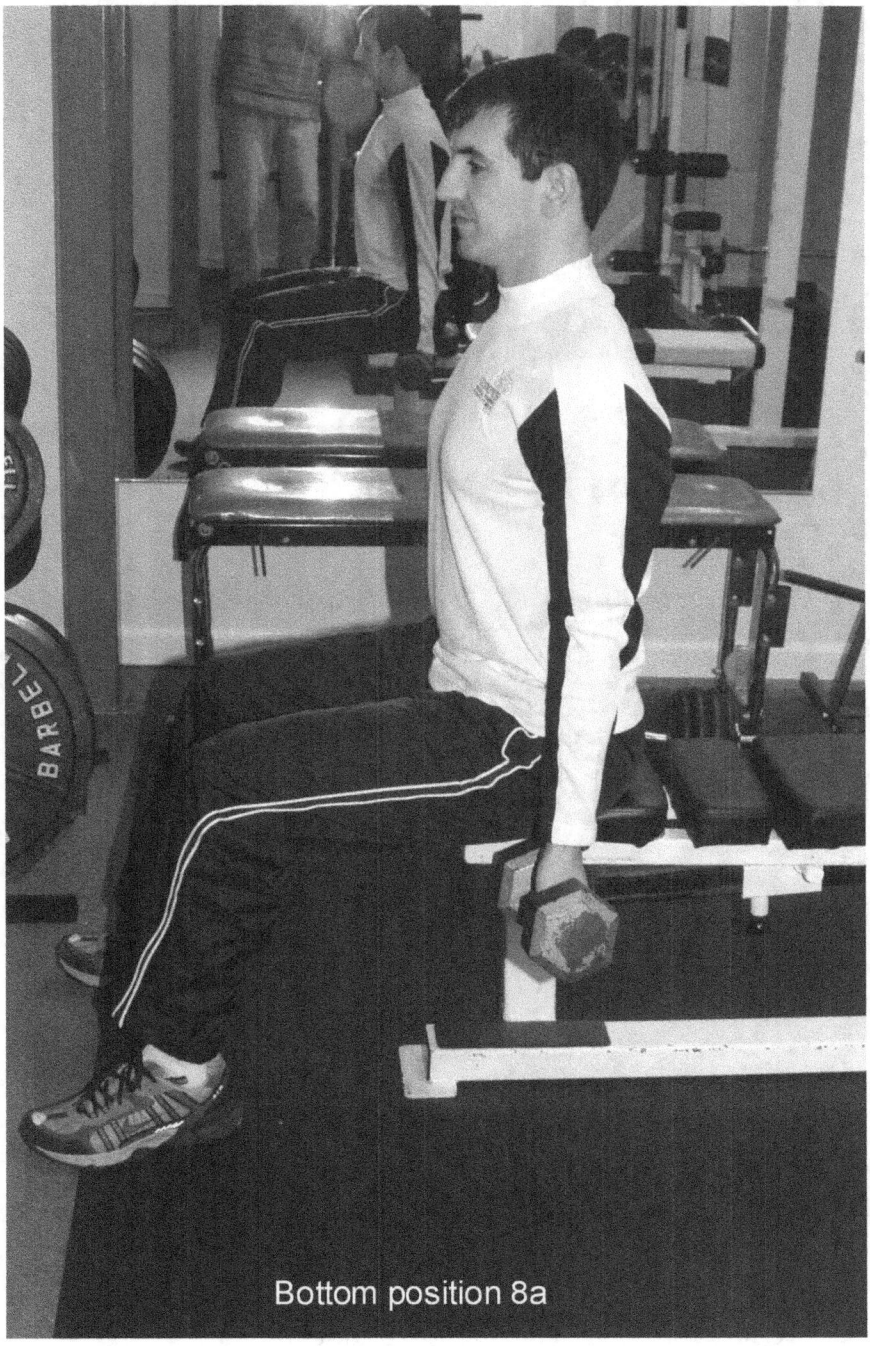

Bottom position 8a

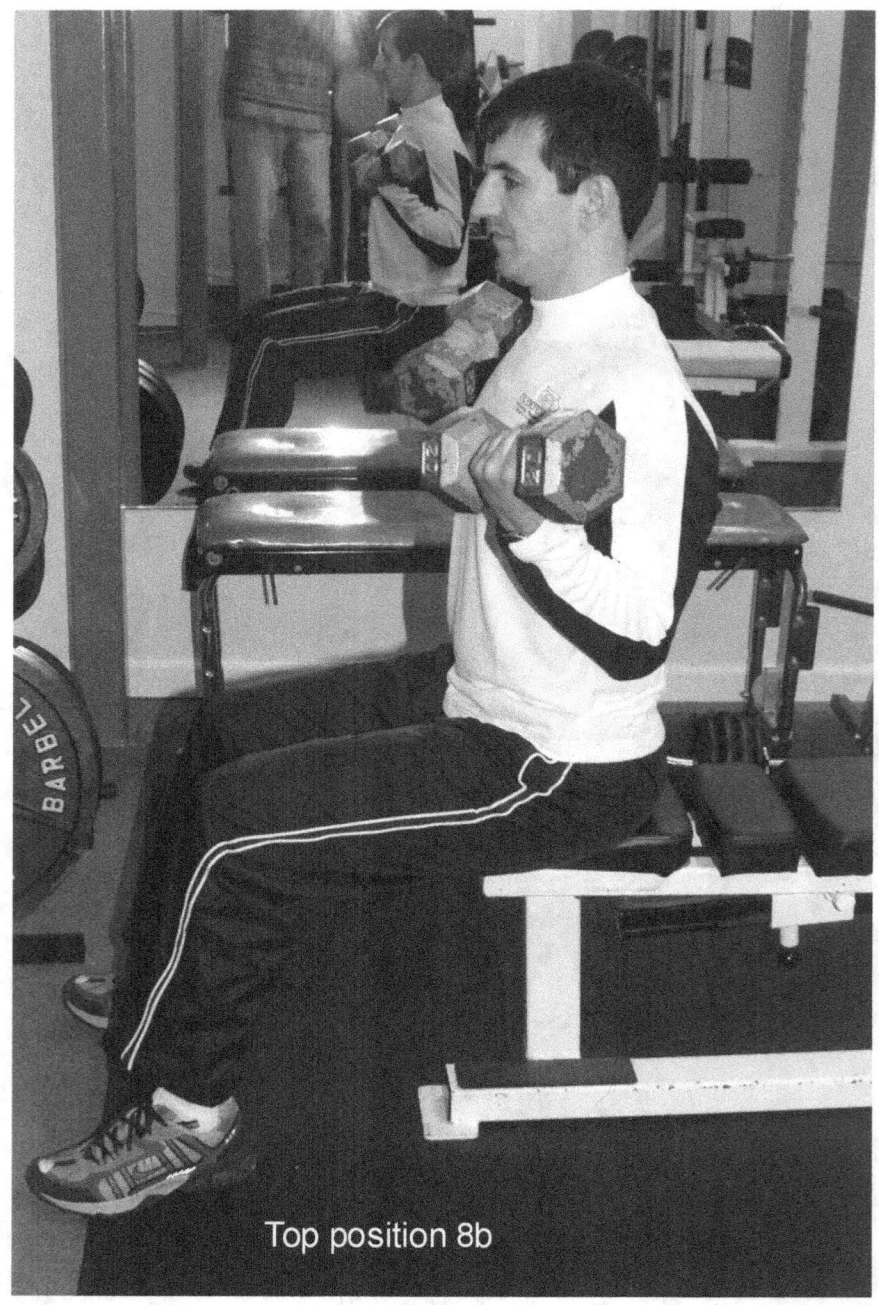

Top position 8b

<u>Main Muscles worked</u>: Biceps (front of arms)
<u>Execution of the Exercise</u>: Refer to pictures 8a, 8b.
1.   Sit at the end of the bench with your legs together. Your arms should

be straight down at your sides with your palms facing forward. Your back should be straight (pictures 8a).

2.   Curl your arms at the elbows but keep the elbows secured to the side and not moving. Stop once your forearms cannot get any closer to the bicep. Do not bend your wrists inward (picture 8b).

3.   Lower arms slowly.

Curls with tubing

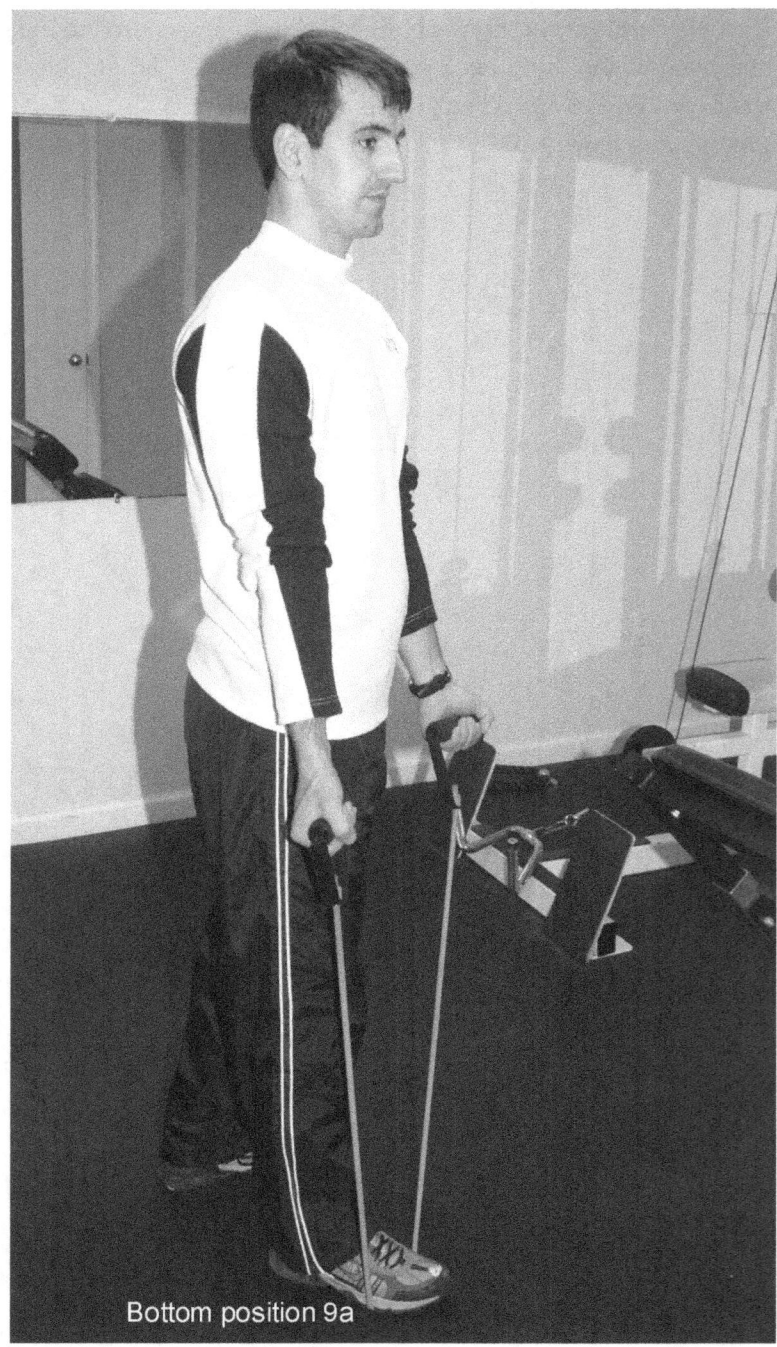

Bottom position 9a

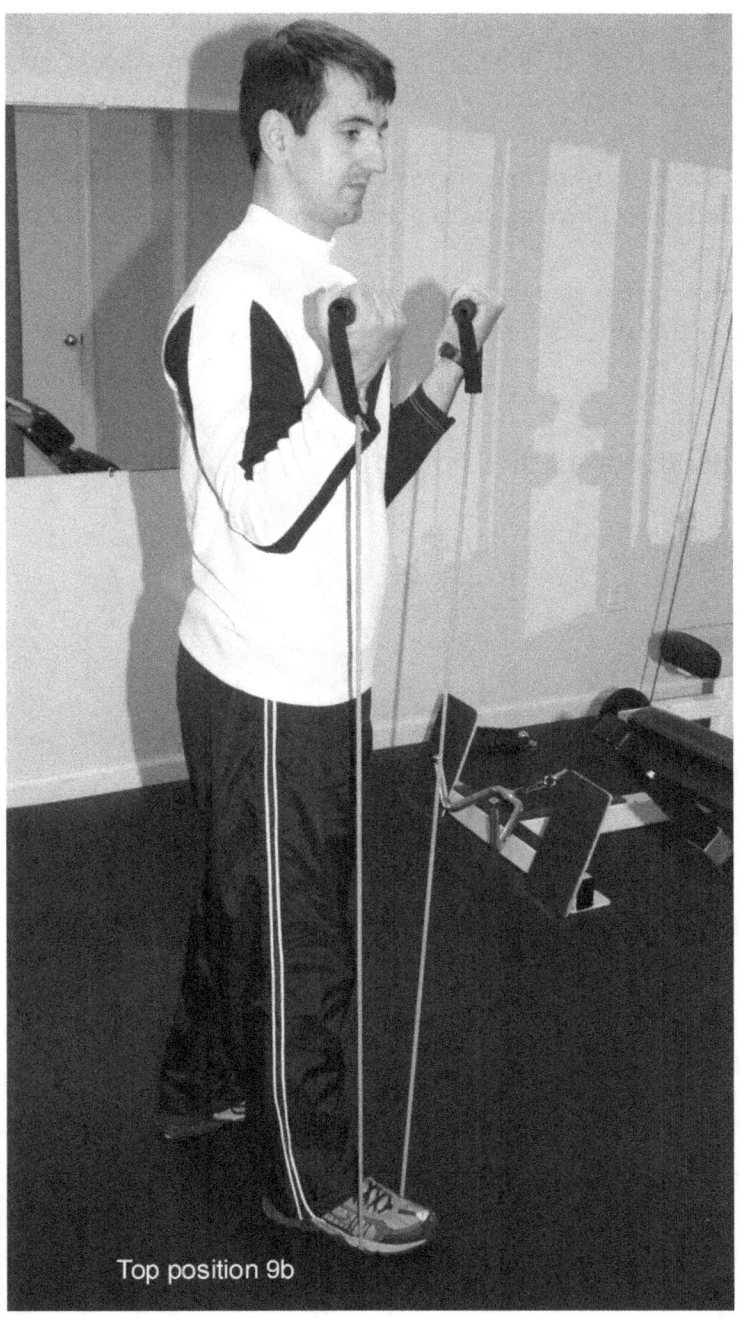

Top position 9b

<u>Main Muscles worked</u>: Biceps (front of arms)
<u>Execution of the Exercise</u>: Refer to pictures 9a, 9b.

1. Begin by stepping on the middle of the tubing on the centerline of your body right in front of you. Your palms should be facing forward, with your elbows at your sides and slightly to the front (picture 9a).

2. Without moving your elbows or bending your wrists, curl your arms until your forearms cannot get any closer to your biceps (picture 9b).

3. Once in the top position lower your arms again nice and slowly remembering not to move your elbows. Repeat the process.

Exercises that work the Triceps (back of the arms)

Triceps overhead extension with tubing

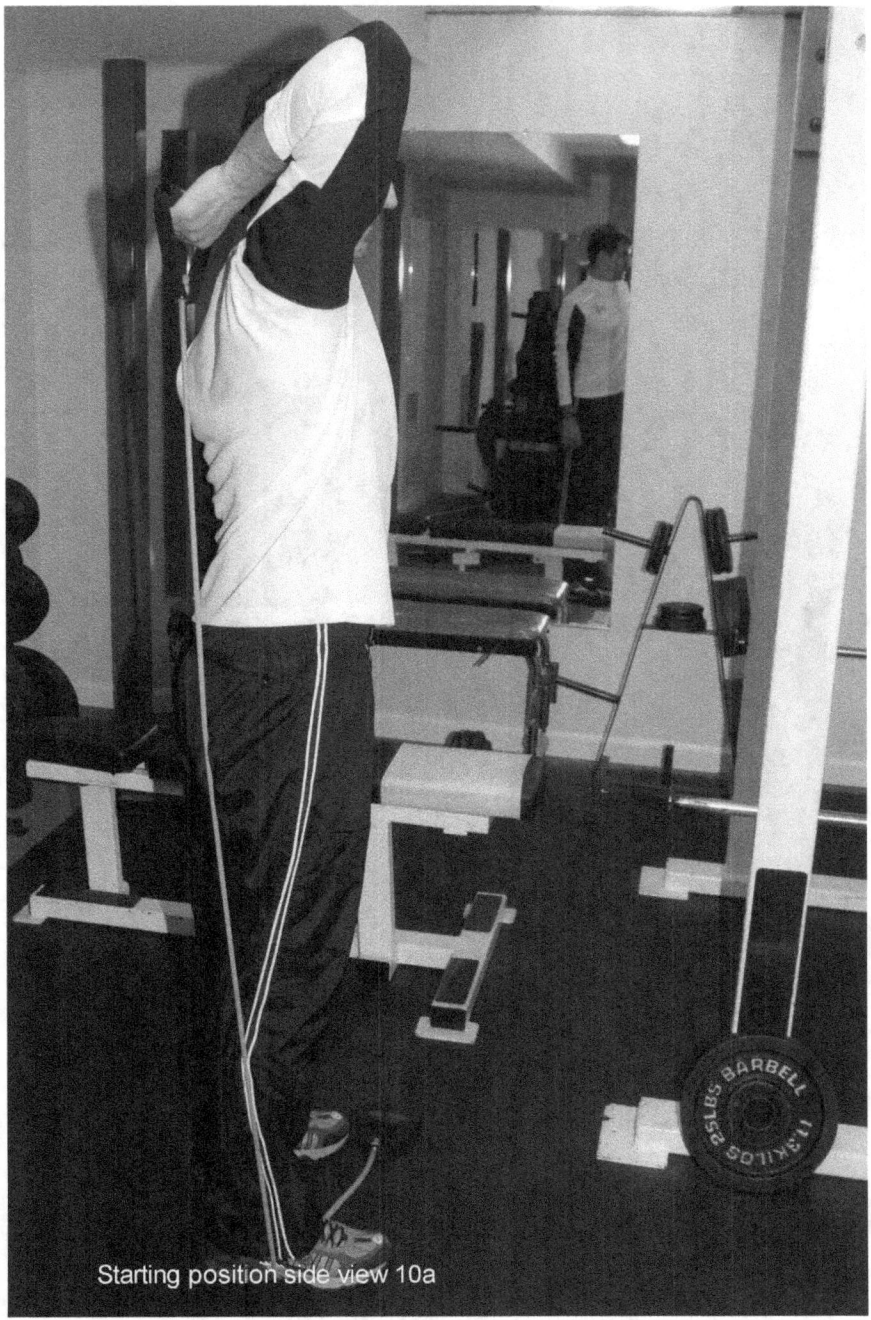

Starting position side view 10a

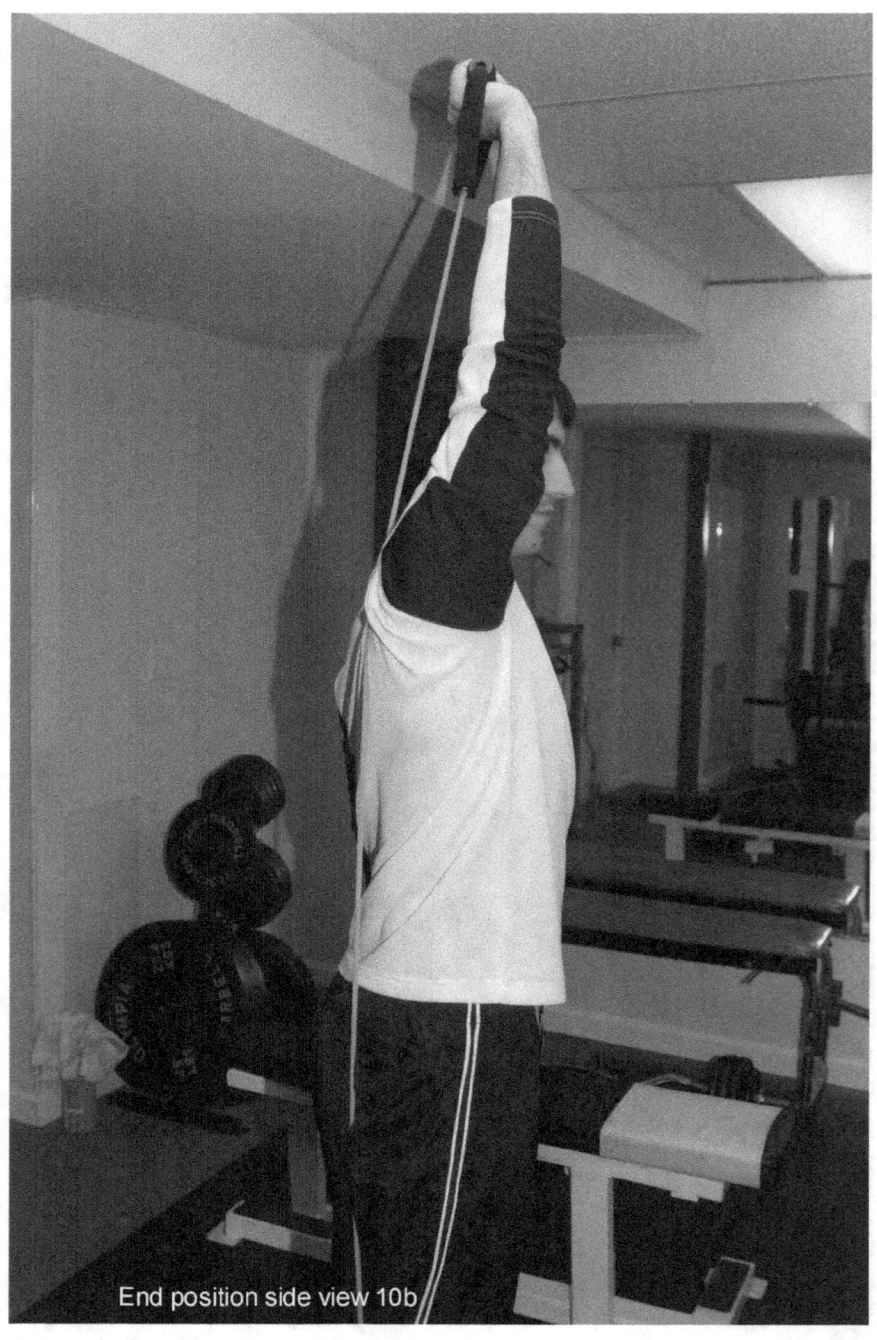

End position side view 10b

<u>Main Muscles worked</u>: Triceps (back of arms)
<u>Execution of the Exercise</u>: Refer to pictures 10a and 10b.

1. Step on one end of the tubing and grab the other end with your hand. Place your elbow overhead with your arm bent backwards (picture 10a).
2. Keeping your elbow in place extend your arms straight overhead (pictures 10b).
3. Once you reach full extension of the arm, lower the arm slowly and repeat the process.

Lying triceps extensions

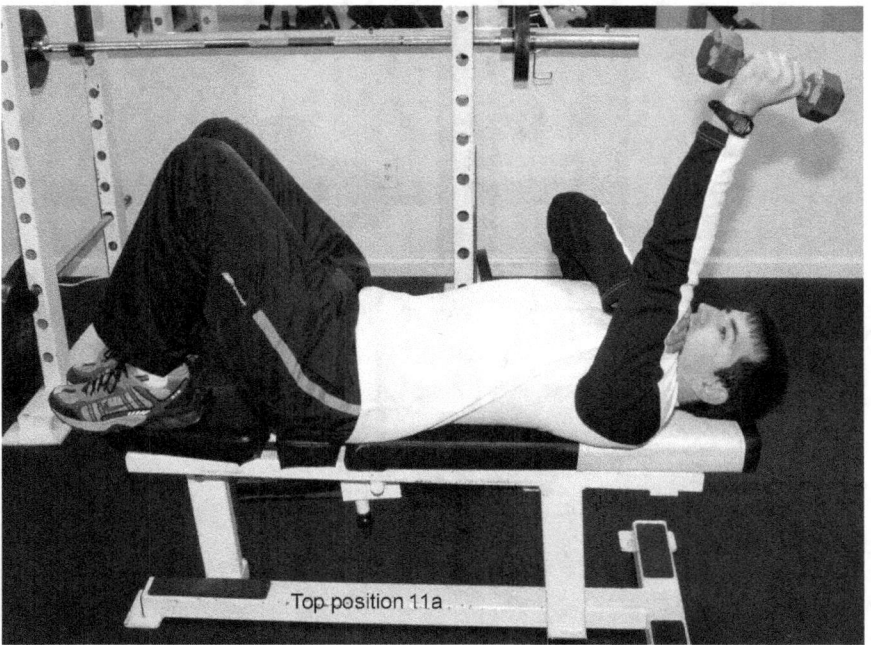

Top position 11a

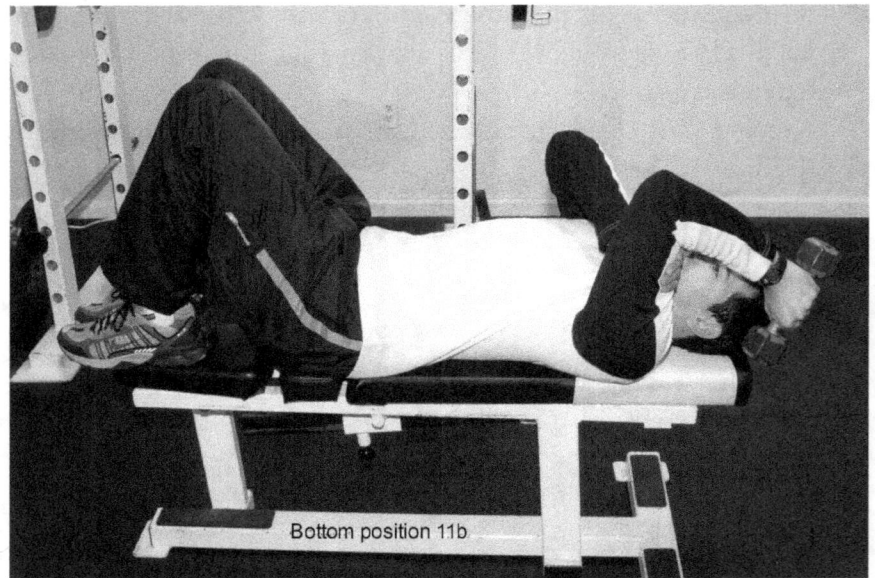

Bottom position 11b

Main Muscles worked: Triceps (back of arms)

Execution of the Exercise: Refer to pictures 11a, 11b.

1. Lie on the bench as in picture 11a. Hold your arm straight and leaning slightly back, with the other hand holding your bicep (picture 20.1a).
2. Bend at the elbow and bring the dumbbell down to your ear. Be careful not to hit your head (picture 11b).

Exercises that work the legs

Dumbbell Squats

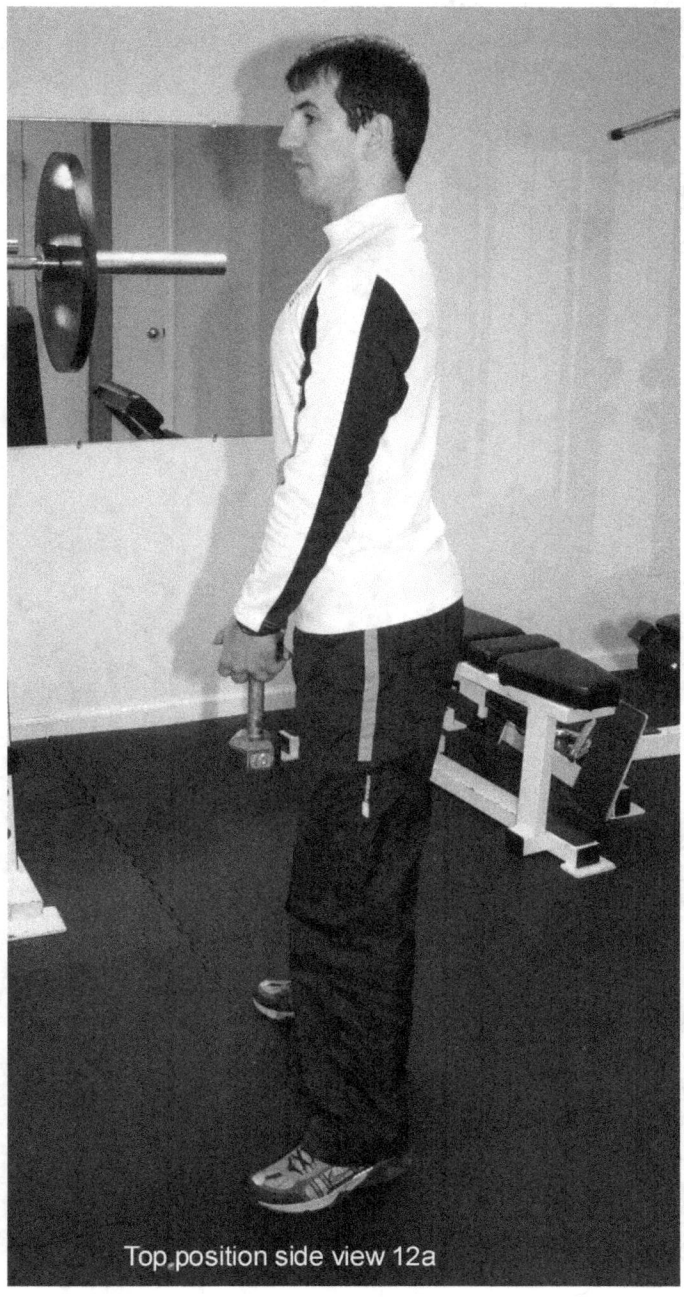

Top position side view 12a

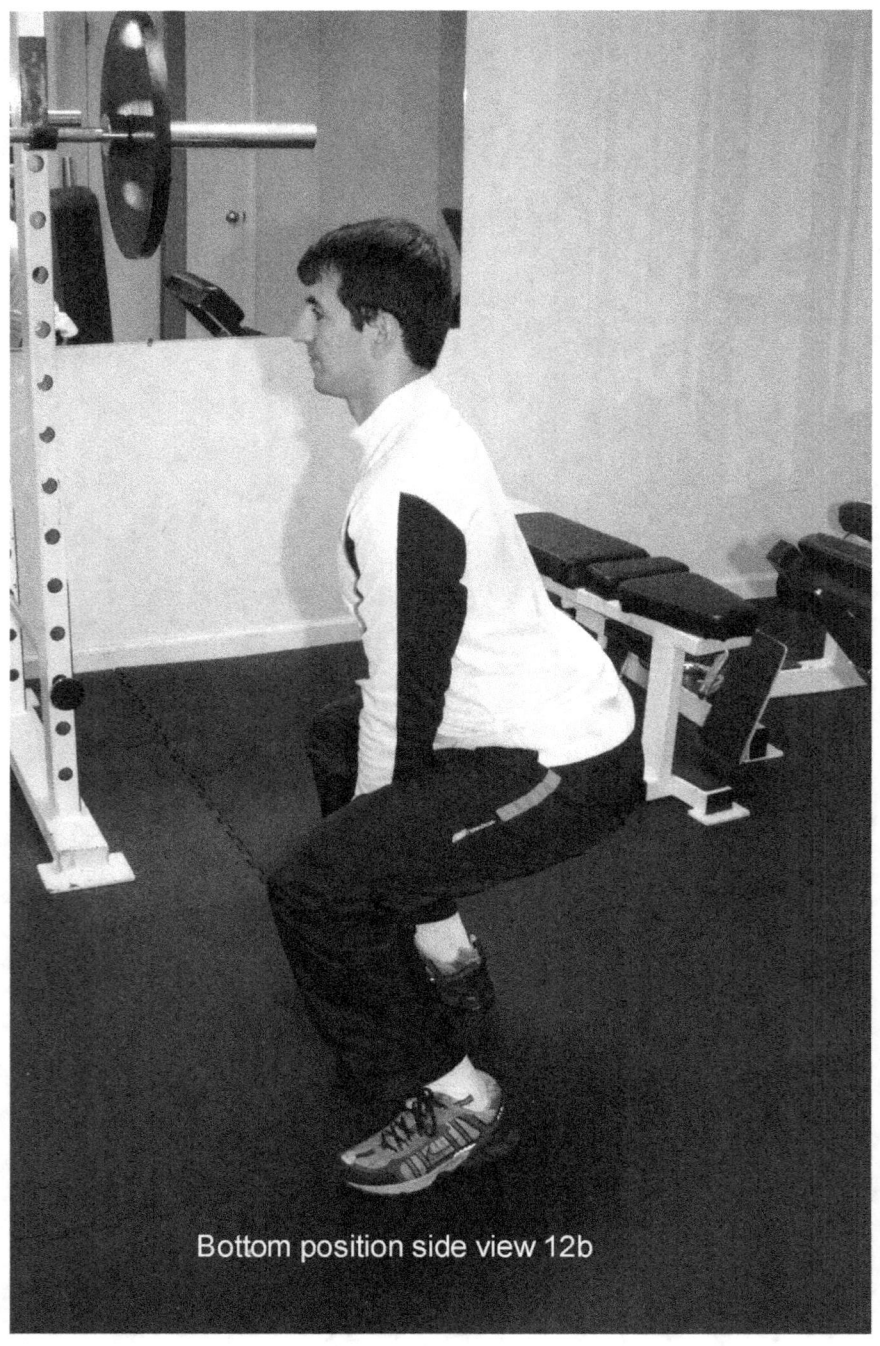

Bottom position side view 12b

Main Muscles worked: Quadriceps, hamstrings, gluteus maximus (front of the thighs, back of the thighs and buttocks).

<u>Execution of the Exercise</u>: Refer to pictures 12a and 12b.

1. Hold the dumbbell between your legs with interlocking fingers. Your feet should be shoulder width apart with toes slightly pointing out (picture 12a).

2. Lower the dumbbell between your legs by bringing your hips down and back. Make sure your spine stays straight and your knees track in the same direction as your toes, but do not go past the toes. Once your thighs are parallel to the ground or slightly higher, stop and go back up (picture 12b).

Note: If it is too difficult for you to squat that low, squat only halfway at the beginning until you get strong enough to go lower.

Holding on Squats

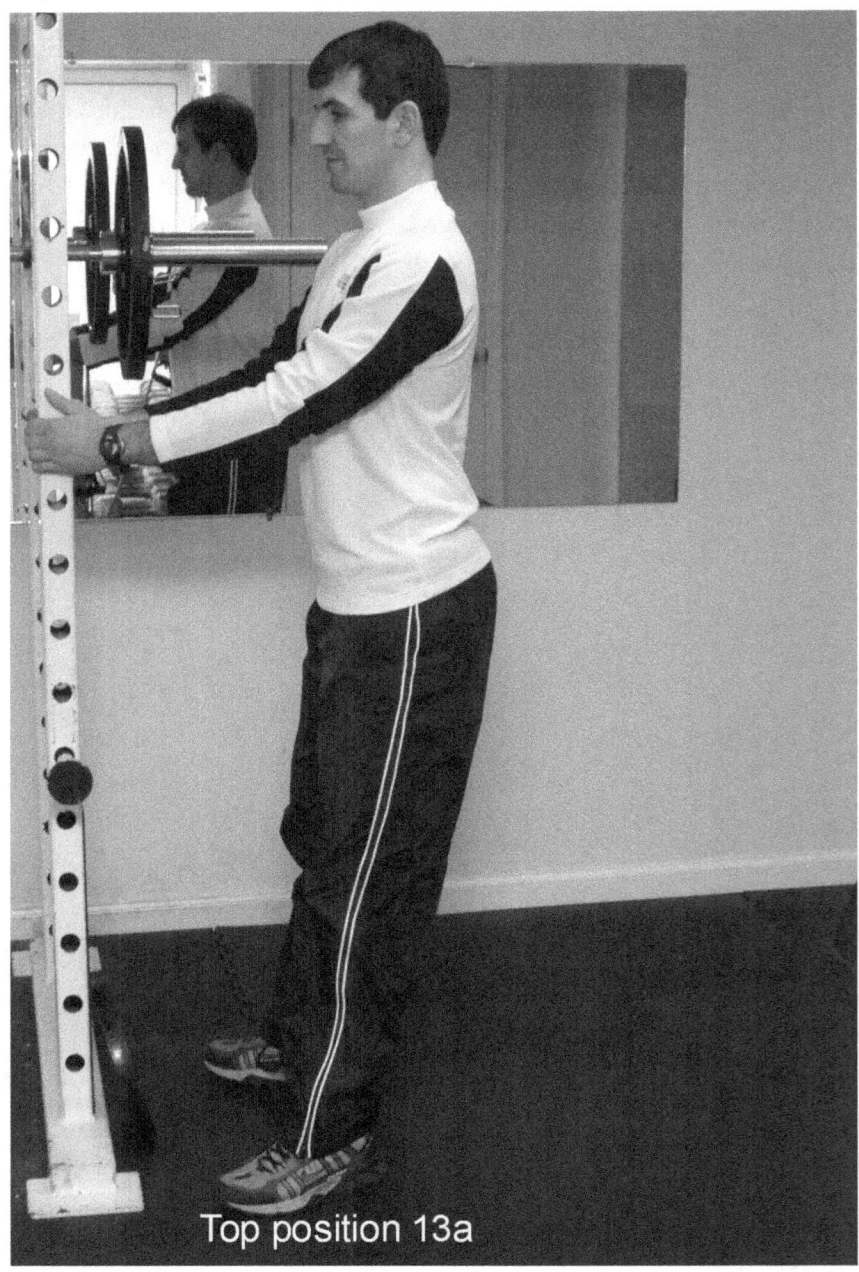

Top position 13a

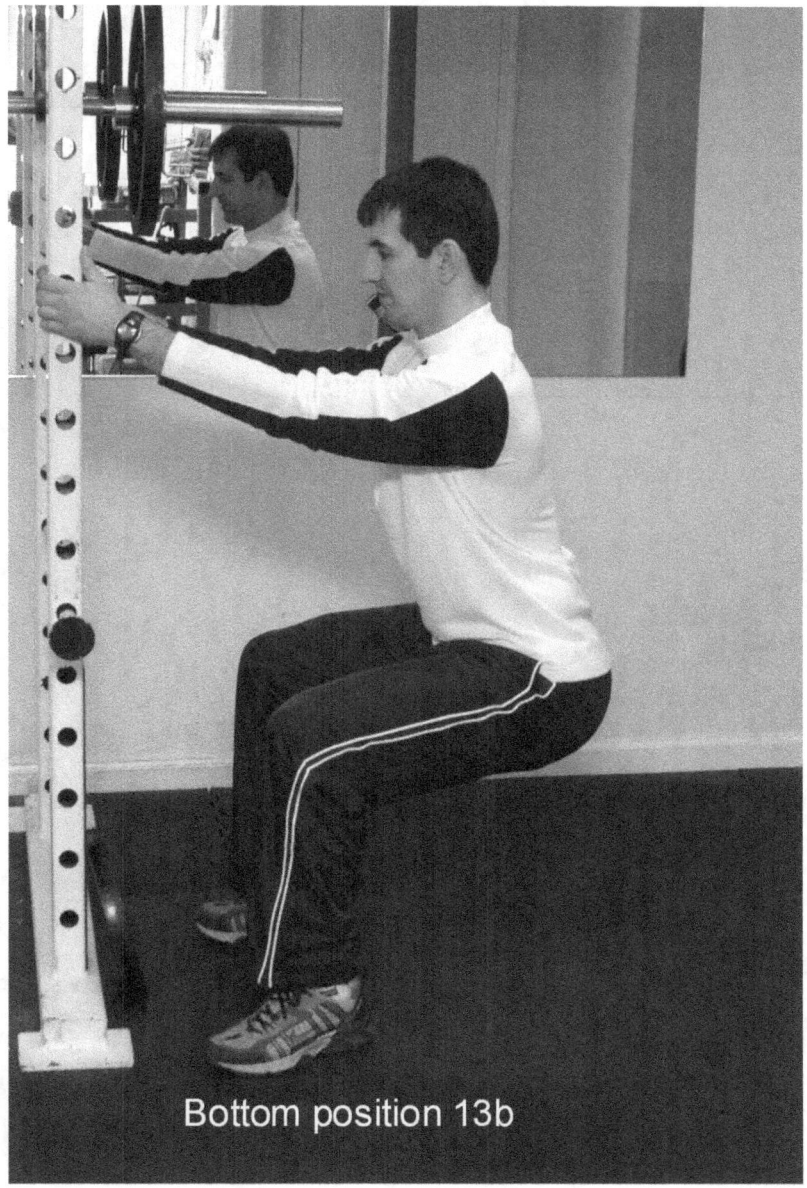

Bottom position 13b

Main Muscles worked: Quadriceps, hamstrings, gluteus maximus (front of the thighs, back of the thighs and buttocks).

Execution of the Exercise: Refer to pictures 13a, 13b.

1.   Stand in front of something you can hold on to and will not fall over, such as a pole. Hold on to the pole at around waist height. Stand

with your feet shoulder width apart and your toes slightly pointing out (picture 13a).

2. Still holding at waist height, move your hips down and back as if you are about to sit on a chair, until your thighs are parallel to the ground. At this point, stop and return to the top position (picture 13b).

Exercises that work the abdominal muscles.

Crunches legs down

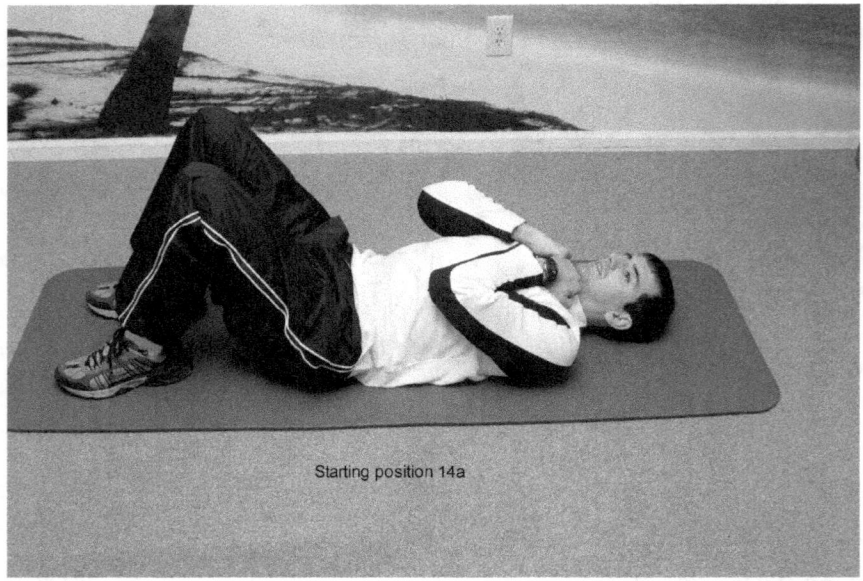

Starting position 14a

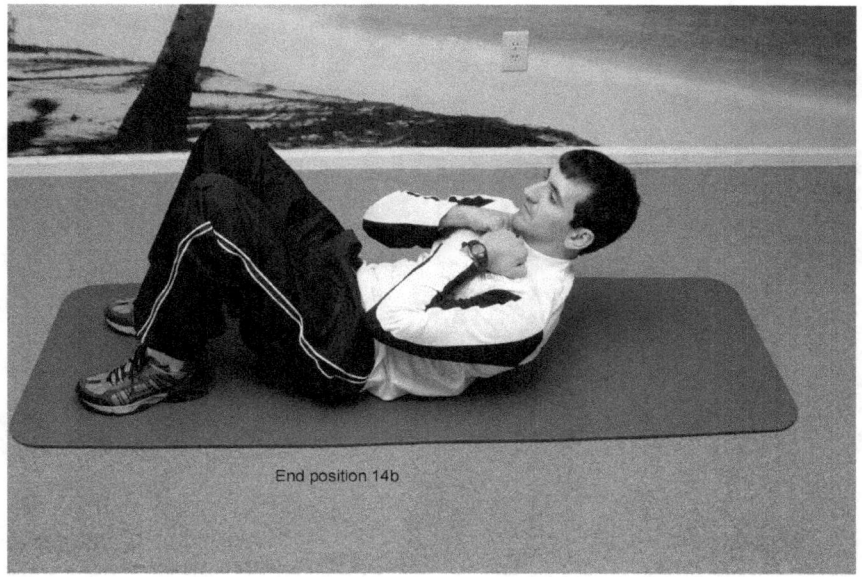

End position 14b

Main Muscles worked: Rectus abdominis (Abs)

Execution of the Exercise: Refer to pictures 14a, 14b.

1. Get into position as shown in picture 14a, keeping your arms against your body and your fists under your chin.

2. When you contract the abs, concentrate on bringing your ribcage closer to the hip. Your shoulder blades should lift off the ground but your lower back should stay on the ground (picture 14b).

3. Once you have reached the end position, lower your body slowly to the starting position again and repeat. Make sure your movements are slow and deliberate.

Note: This is the easiest form of crunches and I advice all beginners to start with them.

Crunches Leg up

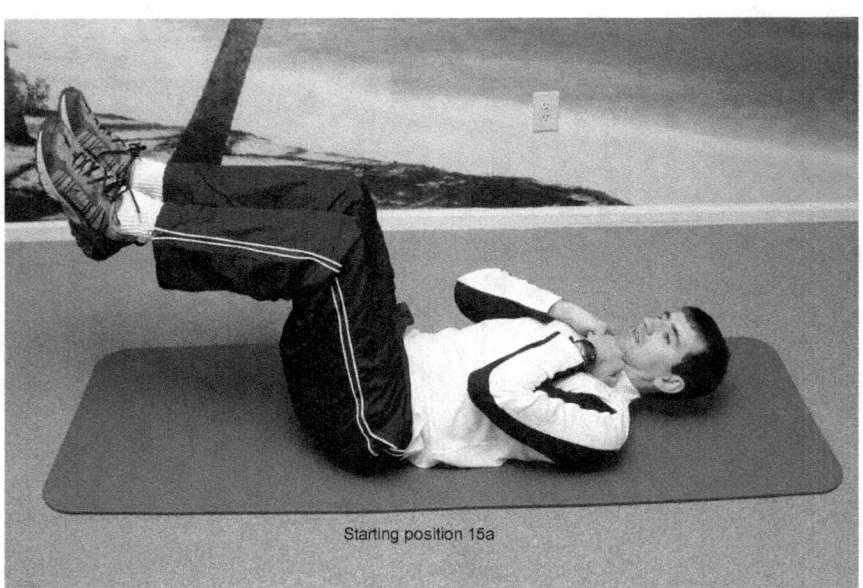

Starting position 15a

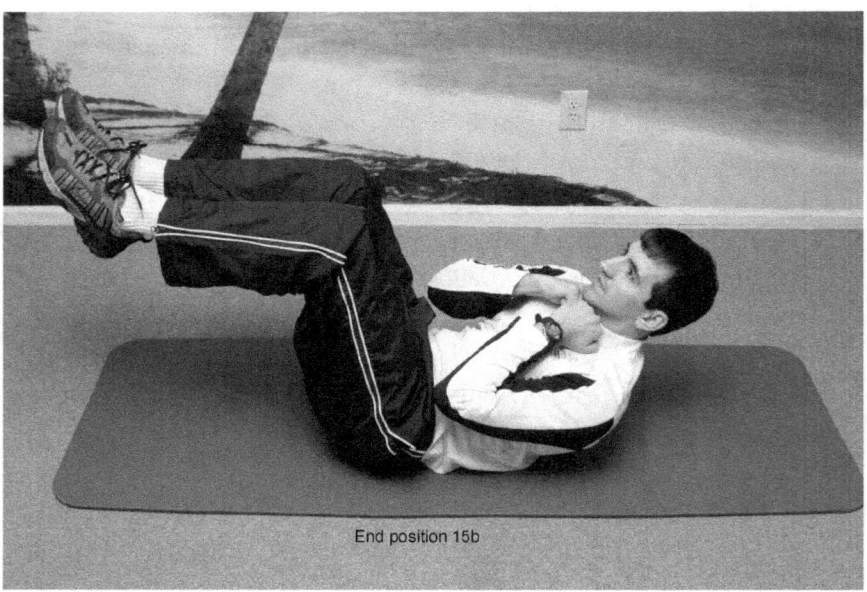

End position 15b

<u>Main Muscles worked</u>: Rectus abdominis (abs)
<u>Execution of the Exercise</u>: Refer to pictures 15a, 15b.

1. Get into the position shown in picture 15a, keeping your arms against your body and your fists under your chin and your legs up.
2. When you contract your abs, concentrate on bringing your ribcage closer to your hips. Your shoulder blades should lift off the ground but your lower back should stay on the ground (picture 15b).
3. Once you have reached the end position, lower your body slowly to the starting point again and repeat. Make sure your movements are slow and deliberate.
4. Make sure that you do not move your legs throughout the crunch.

Note: When crunches with legs down get easy, you should move to these churches.

Exercises that work the lower back

Floor hyperextensions

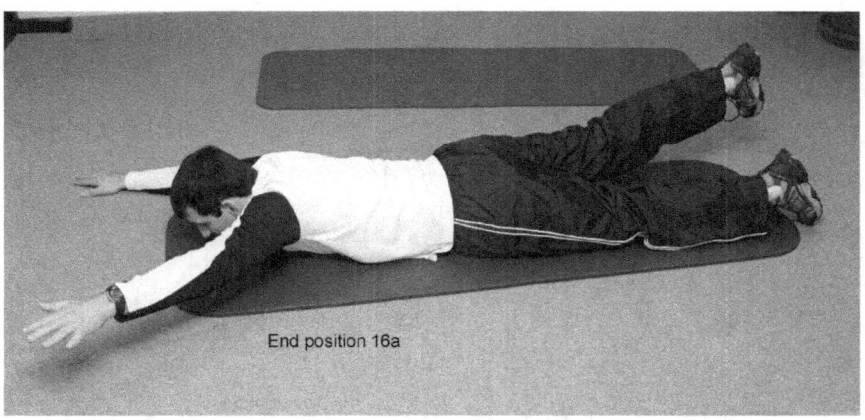

End position 16a

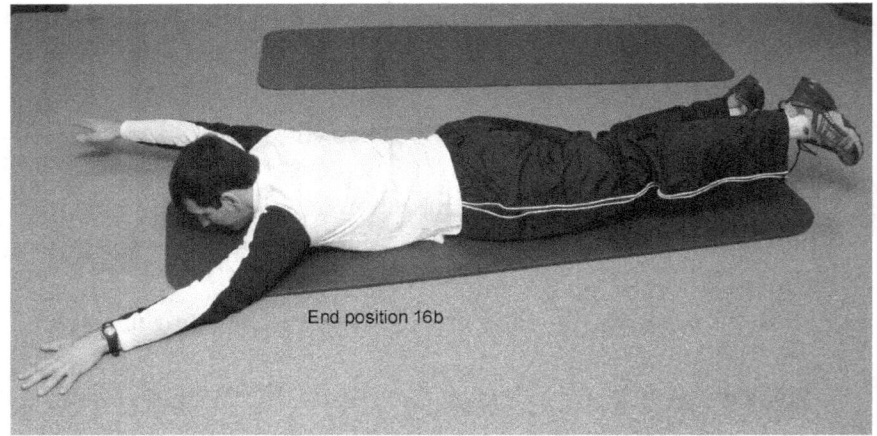

End position 16b

Main Muscles worked: Erector spinae (lower back)

Execution of the Exercise: Refer to pictures 16a and 16b.

1. Start by lying on the floor, on your stomach with both arms over your head.
2. Raise one hand and the opposite leg and keep alternating as in pictures 16a and 16b. Do not raise your hands or legs too high.

Note: This is the easiest way to start strengthening your lower back.

Hyperextension with ball

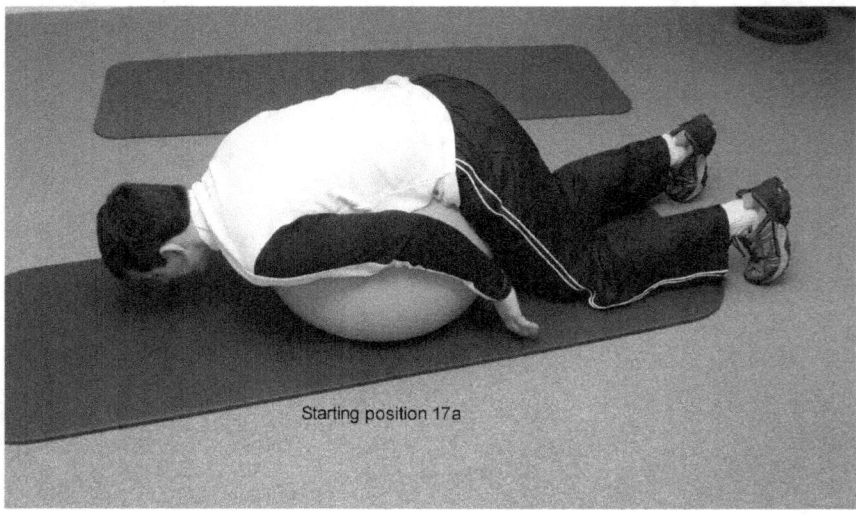

Starting position 17a

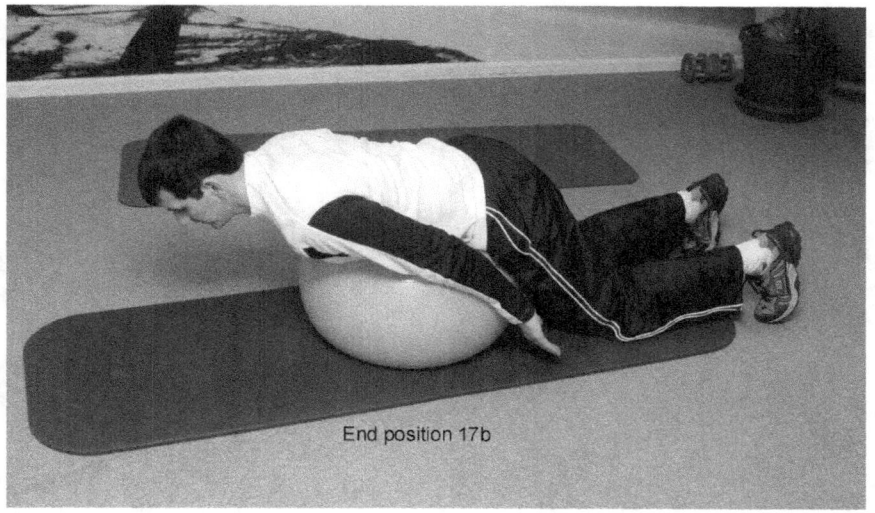

End position 17b

<u>Main Muscles worked</u>: Erector spinae (lower back)
<u>Execution of the Exercise</u>: Refer to pictures 17a, 17b.

1. Place your stomach on the ball and lean over it as in picture 17a. Keep your knees on the ground and your hands at your side.
2. Raise your upper body to a straight position as in picture 17b and repeat.

***

Stretches

Chest stretching

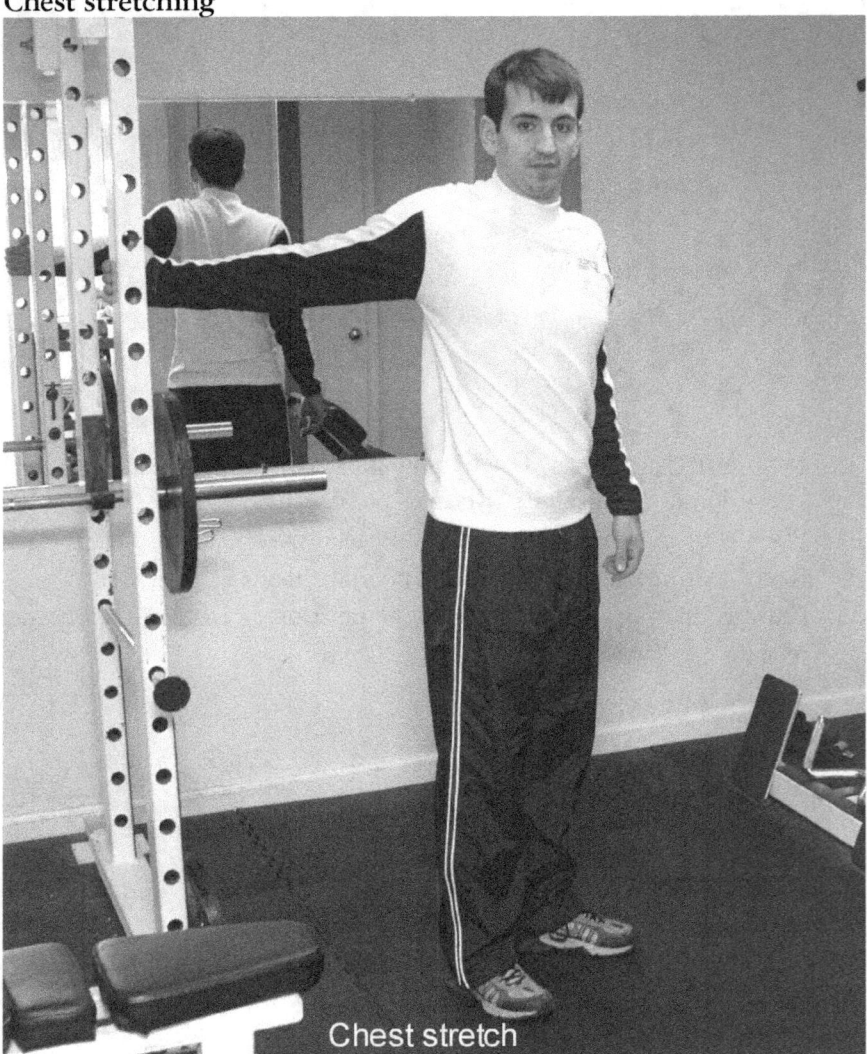

Chest stretch

With your palm facing forward and arm straight, turn your body away from the straight arm to feel the stretch on the chest.

Back stretch

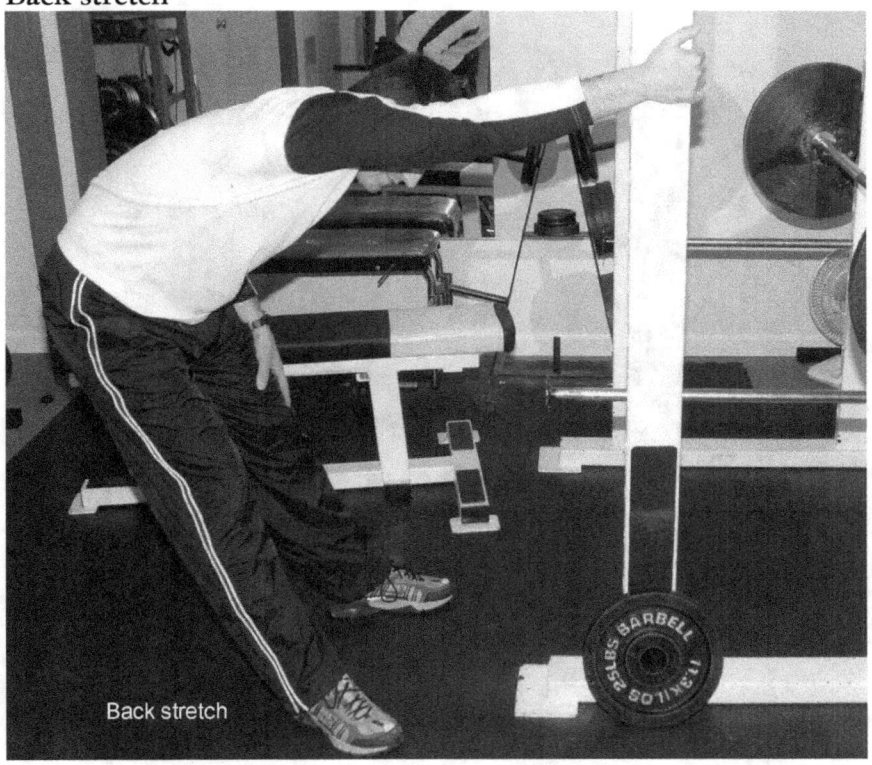

Back stretch

Grab something sturdy, lean backwards, and turn your hips away from the arm that is holding on.

Shoulder stretch

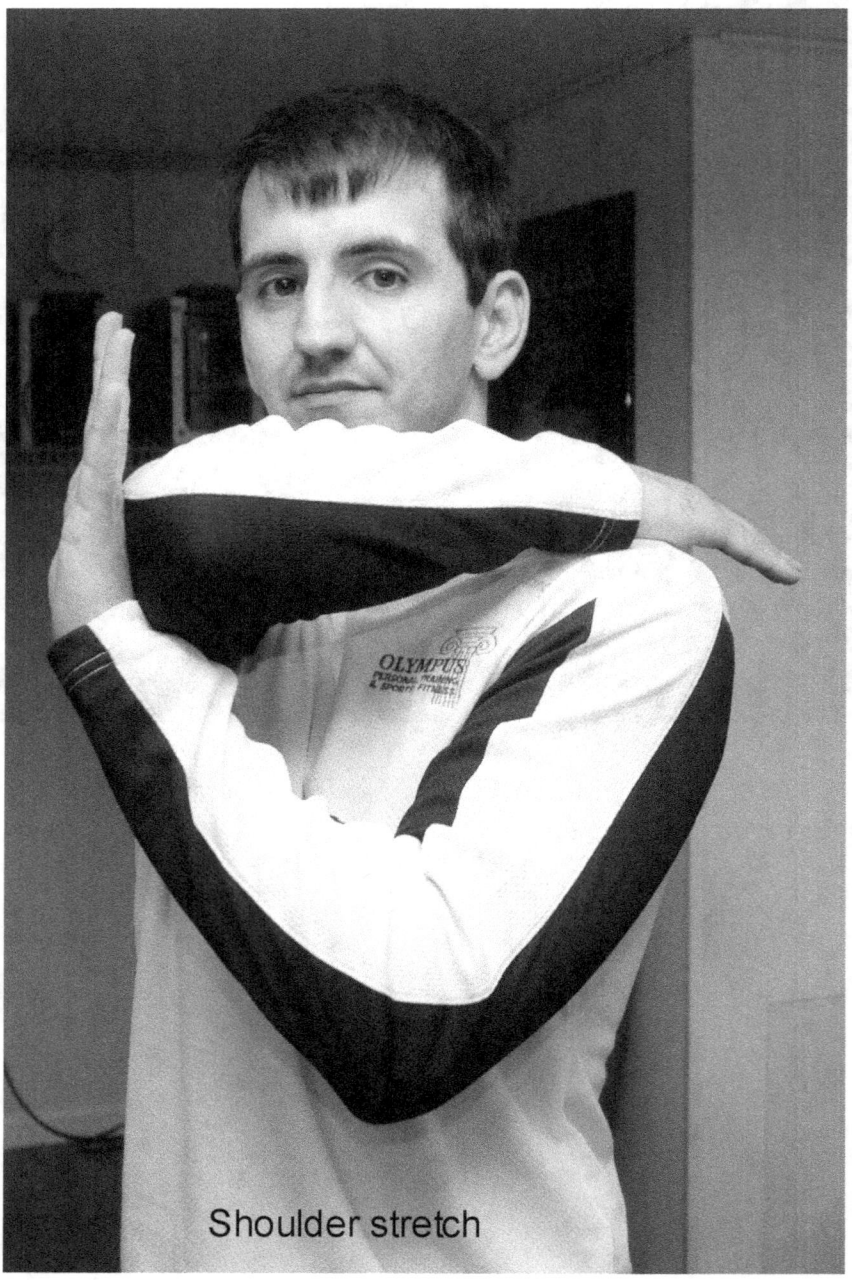

Shoulder stretch

Front view   Pull your elbow towards your chin.

Bicep stretch

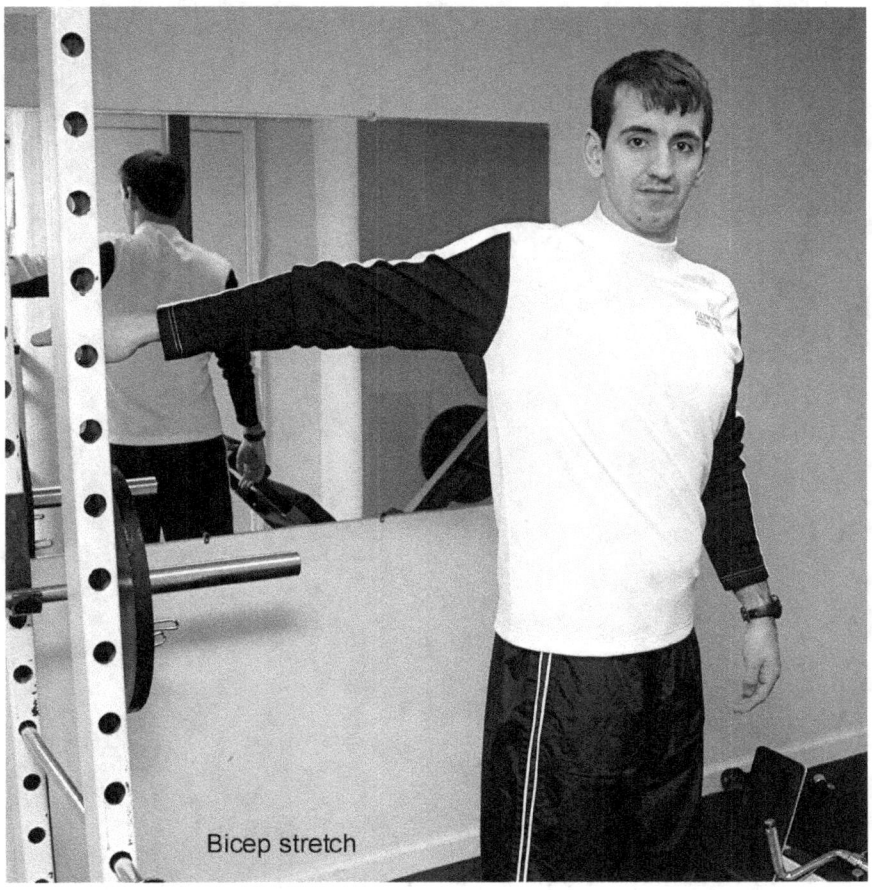

Bicep stretch

With your palm facing down and arm straight, turn your body away from the straight arm to feel the stretch on your biceps.

Triceps Stretch

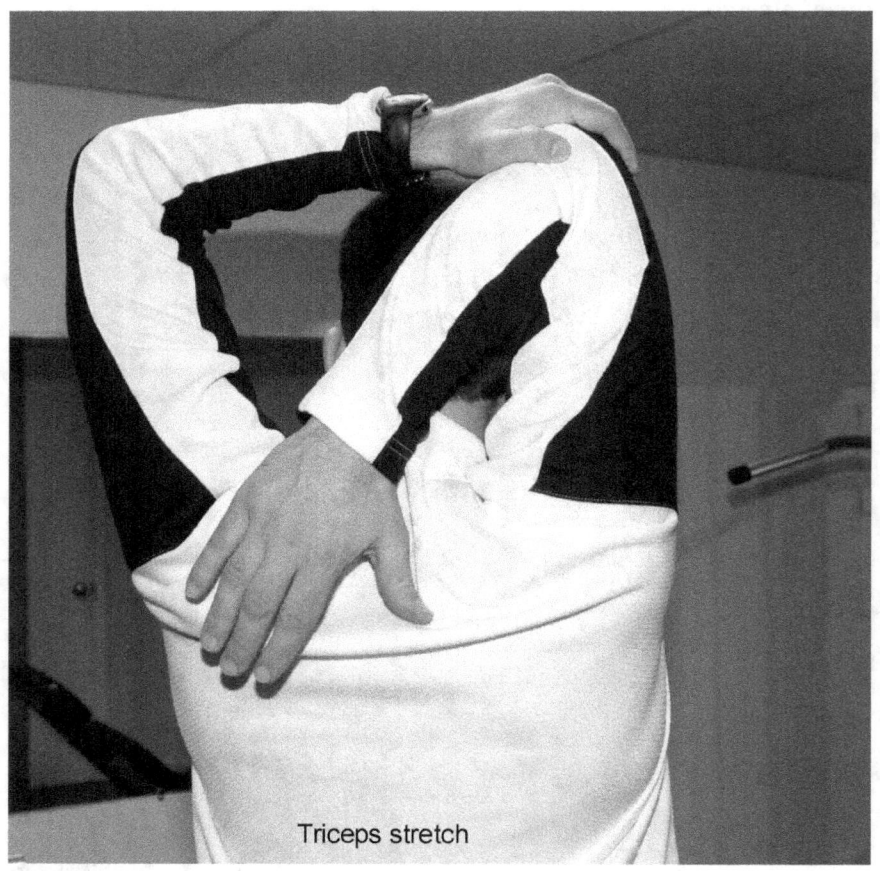

Triceps stretch

Grab your elbow and pull it towards the back of your neck.

Hamstring stretch

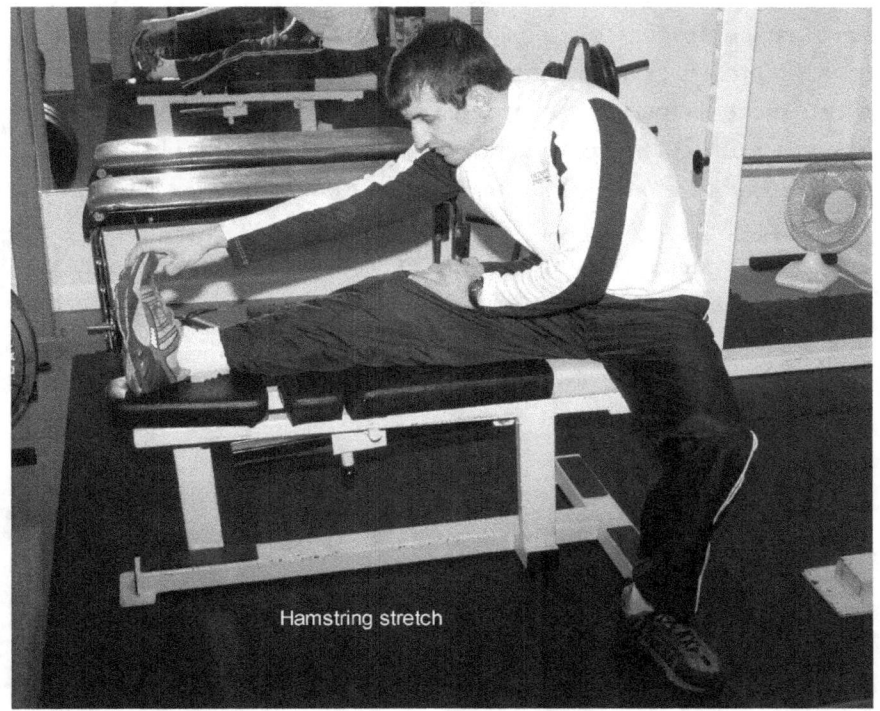

Hamstring stretch

Keeping your leg straight, lean on your leg.

Note:
1. Make sure you repeat the stretches on both sides.
2. Make sure you hold each stretch for at least 10 to 20 seconds.
3. Do each stretch right after the exercise.

Aerobic Exercises

Before starting any exercise program, make sure you get clearance from your doctor. If you have any knee or foot problems, make sure you talk to your doctor about what type of aerobics would be best for you.

Walking: Walking is the best aerobic exercise you can start with, unless your doctor has told you not to walk because of major knee problems or other problems. Walking is low impact and low intensity exercise, which makes it perfect for beginners. It is also easy to do anywhere. You can walk outside or you can walk on a treadmill. The difference between walking on a treadmill instead of outside is that treadmill is lower impact and you have the option of inclining it to increase the intensity without increasing the impact. For some people, however, the treadmill is boring. Putting a TV in front of the treadmill might solve this problem. If you want to walk outside, walk on grass or on a track. If this is not available, walk on a dirt road. Walking on the pavement should be your last choice.

Jogging: Jogging is the next step up from walking. Because jogging is higher impact than walking, do not jog everyday. Take a break between jogs, especially if you are a beginner.

Running: If you are a beginner, do not run until you have been jogging for at least six months and you do not have any knee problems.

Elliptical: The elliptical machine is a great way to do your aerobics. It allows you to do high intensity aerobics with very little impact on your knees.

Stepper: The stepper is another great aerobic machine that allows you to do high intensity aerobics with little impact on your knees. However, just because there is low impact on the knees does not mean there is no strain on the knees. The stepper might make certain knee problems worse. If you have knee problems, consult your doctor first before doing any aerobic exercises.
Note: Do not lean over the stepper. Keep your body straight.

Swimming: This is the lowest impact exercise you can do, and it is perfect for the significantly overweight person who would like to get some aerobic training without worrying whether their knees will be able to take the extra impact. The only negative aspect about swimming when it come to weight loss (fat loss) is that for some reason, your body does not burn fat the same way as it would when you do an aerobic exercise on dry land. It is believed that this is because your body needs the fat to isolate it from the water and to keep the body afloat better. By the way, these are theories. I think swimming is a great aerobic exercise for the significantly overweight, at least to start with, because of the low impact on the knees. Later as you lose some weight, you can pick a low impact aerobic exercise on dry land, such as the elliptical, stepper, or bike.

Biking: Biking or using a stationary bike is a great aerobic exercise. It is low impact so it is excellent for greatly overweight people.

Other Aerobic Exercises: You get considerable aerobic benefits from any exercise or sport that keeps your heart rate over 60% of its maximum constantly for at least 20 minutes. Of course, you get health benefits and weight loss benefits from any activity no matter how short the activity.

CHAPTER 6

Jump Start Your Weight Loss the Healthy Way

Many weight loss products and programs promise fast weight loss. Most of them don't deliver what they promise, and the ones that do compromise your health. I always put health over weight loss, because what is the point of having a nice body if you do not have your health? The method that I will describe to you in this chapter is not just going to help speed up your weight loss for three to four weeks, but is actually good for your health and body. The reason this way of eating is so good is that besides helping you lose between 12 to 20 pounds in four weeks, it will also help detoxify your body. I recommend doing this type of diet for two to four weeks at a time, and aim to do it three to four times a year even after you have achieved your target weight. This, by the way, is not a new diet; a similar eating regimen has been practiced by Orthodox Christians during Lent and three other times each year for hundreds of years. Recent research has revealed that there are great health benefits to eating this way. The average weight loss that I have observed in people is three to five pounds per week, during the course of the first three to four weeks on this eating regimen. Weight loss does slow down after the first four weeks. Notice there is no fine print "results not typical" or "results may vary" because this is the average weight loss per week, not the exception. My advice is to eat this way for two to four weeks in a row, four to five times a year. You can also eat like this one to two days per week throughout the year to keep your body detoxified and help you with your weight loss efforts. Even when you reach your goal, it is not a bad idea to continue to do this kind of regimen. If you want to lose some weight quickly and still stay healthy, try this eating pattern. You will be pleasantly surprised at the results, but don't just take my word for it; try it for yourself.

The Eating Regimen

The eating regimen is very simple, although keep in mind that in the beginning it will be a little hard to get used to eating this way. It does get easier over time. I know this firsthand because I have done it myself and I do it every year. Remember, nothing worthwhile comes without some sacrifice, and after you see the results on your body and energy levels, you will definitely think it worth the sacrifice.

The following are the only foods you should eat during the duration of this program:

1. All the vegetables you want (cooked and uncooked). Be careful what you put on the vegetables, no creamy dressings of any kind and no butter. Keep any sauce you use low fat and low sodium.
2. All the fruits you want (raw only).
3. One to two servings of beans per day.
4. You can have all soy products (soymilk, tofu, soy cheese, etc.).
5. Eat one to two servings of fish or egg whites per week.
6. Eat one ounce of seeds or nuts per day.
7. No more than two servings of "best starches." Check the Food List in the appendix of this workbook to see what I consider best starches. Note: The less starch you eat, the more weight you will lose.
8. Take a multi-vitamin.

The following are foods you should not eat during the duration of this program:

1. All animal products and their byproducts (meat, chicken, eggs, dairy products, butter, etc.).
2. All junk food and refined food. To see what I consider junk and refined foods, see the Food List in the appendix of this book under "Foods to avoid like the plague."

During this time, you will be eating a high vegetable diet. You will be surprised not only by how much weight you can lose eating this way, but also at how great you will feel and how energized you will become. For some people it is very hard to eat this way for a long time. Although

I recommend eating this way for at least two weeks, you will still reap the benefits doing it for shorter periods such as three to four days or even one to two days. For maximum weight loss, do it for three to four weeks and then follow my regular diet recommendations, which you will find in Step 4 of Chapter 3. Again, do not just take my word for it; try it for yourself and see the results first hand.

Always talk to your doctor before trying any diet or exercise program.

Suggestions to help you with your eating

Food should be viewed as fuel for the body, not as entertainment; so you should always judge food by the quality of fuel it provides your body and not just by how good it tastes.

- Keep easily prepared vegetables in the house.
- Keep fruits that you like in the house at all times.
- Make a list of food that should always be in the house.
- Look up vegetable recipes and try them out.
- Don't keep white flour products around the house.
- Don't keep junk/refined food around the house.
- Keep your foods low fat. Try not to use fatty dressings and sauces on your food even if it is a good fat such as olive oil or flax seed oil. You only need small amounts of the essential oils.
- Every weekend, plan your meals for the week ahead and make sure you have all the ingredients you need.
- Get into the habit of bringing your own food to work.
- Many vegetable dishes can be precooked and eaten cold. Try some.
- Look up some good low fat fish recipes.
- Look up some good low fat bean/legume recipes.
- Double or triple the vegetable servings per meal and make the meat portion smaller.
- A meal does not have to have meat or starch to be called a meal.
- Consider switching to soy products such as soymilk.
- Don't be afraid to check out new recipes. Check out Healthy Recipes in the appendix of this workbook.

You will be surprised at how easy it is to eat healthy!

Sample Menus

Note: *As you will notice, I do not give portion sizes for each meal. The reason is that no one can really tell you the exact number of calories your body needs, all the formulas you see that help you figure out how many calories your body needs are only estimates. The best way to figure out how much food you should eat is to listen to your body and go by how you feel. Eat only when you are hungry (true hunger, not a craving), and eat until you have satisfied your hunger but are not overfull. Try to have set times when you eat each day, even when you are snacking. Keep in mind the main reason you should be eating is to nourish your body. The better your body is nourished, the better it will function and the faster you will lose the excess fat your body is holding.*

Sample menu 1
Breakfast: Any fruit
Lunch: Big salad with any kind of vegetables on it, with a low fat dressing
Dinner: Spinach & Rice (see recipes)
Snack Choices: Nuts, seeds, fruits, baby carrots, and bell peppers

Sample menu 2
Breakfast: Any fruit, glass of soymilk.
Lunch: Sushi with fish, a side salad, low fat or no fat dressing.
Dinner: Ratatouille (see recipes)
Snack Choices: Nuts, seeds, fruit salad, baby carrots, bell peppers

Sample menu 3
Breakfast: Whole grain high fiber cold cereal with soymilk
Lunch: Veggie burger on whole grain bread with lettuce, tomato, onions,
and a small salad. Use a low fat or no fat dressing.
Dinner: Mediterranean-style Lima Beans (see recipes)
Snack Choices: Nuts, seeds, fruits, baby carrots. bell peppers

Sample menu 4

Breakfast: Fruit

Lunch: Salmon with double vegetables, small salad, low fat or no fat dressing.

Dinner: Eggplant and Beans with Tomato Salad, Greek style (see recipes)

Snack Choices: Nuts, seeds, fruits, baby carrots, and bell peppers

Sample menu 5

Breakfast: Fruits

Lunch: Black-Eyed Pea Salad (see recipe)

Dinner: Artichoke Hearts with Peas (see recipe)

Snack Choices: Nuts, seeds, fruits, baby carrots, and bell peppers

Sample menu 6

Breakfast: Fruits, few almonds

Lunch: Cannelini Bean Salad (see recipe)

Dinner: Peas & Corn with Boiled Chicory Salad (see recipes)

Snack Choices: Nuts, seeds, fruits, baby carrots, and bell peppers

CHAPTER 7

How to maintain your lean and healthy body!

You have achieved the body of your dreams! Now what?

What is the point of achieving a lean and healthy body if you are not going to maintain it? In this program, we leave nothing to chance. We are not satisfied just to see you achieve a lean and healthy body; we want you to be able to maintain it for life. This chapter is dedicated to help you do just that.

Maintenance

By the time you achieve your goal weight, your diet should be excellent and you should have established a good workout and activity routine. Remember, you do not have to be perfect to maintain your weight loss. Keep in mind the 80/20 rule. As long as you do the right things 80% of the time, what you do the other 20% of the time will not have much impact on your weight and health (excluding, of course, substance abuse).

Proper Nutrition

To help you stay on track with your eating habits, keep reminding yourself that food is fuel, and the better the quality of the fuel you put into your body, the better your body will look, function and feel. I suggest that as a mental exercise you repeat the following phrase to yourself at least 10 times every day for at least four weeks:

"Food is fuel; the better the quality of the fuel I put into my body, the better my body will look, function, and feel."

Memorize this phrase; write it down if you have to. Once you have this embedded in your mind, you will have absolutely no problem avoiding the "bad foods" and reaching for the good ones. Having some "bad food" on occasion is fine, and there is nothing wrong with it. If you have the occasional cookie or cake, enjoy it and do not feel guilty about it. Remember the 80/20 rule. I also recommend that every three to four months, even if you are maintaining your weight with no problem, you follow the eating recommendations for the *Jump Start Program* in Chapter 6 of this book for one to two weeks. It is a great way to detoxify your body and to keep you on track. It is not a bad idea, either, to eat like this for one to two days a week. It is a great way to keep your body not just lean but healthy also. At least once per week read my Diet Recommendations in this program. This will help you maintain good eating habits.

Exercising

As far as exercise goes, it should not be a problem keeping it up, especially the resistance training part. You can cut down on your aerobic exercising a bit if you like, because now that you only need to maintain your weight you do not need to do as much. If you decide to cut down the amount of aerobics you do per week, cut it down one day at a time. In other words if, for example, you were doing six aerobic workouts per week, cut down to five and stay there for at least two weeks. If your weight stays the same after the two weeks and you would like to cut your aerobics further, that is fine: you can cut down to four days per week. If you find that your weight goes up, you might want to reconsider or maybe look at your eating habits more carefully. Remember, the more you exercise, the more forgiving your diet can be. Because everybody is different and diet is a key factor in your weight, I cannot tell you how much or how little aerobics you need to do to maintain your weight. You will need to experiment and find out for yourself.

What I can tell you is that you need to do at least three aerobic workouts per week, of at least 20 minutes each, to enable you to maintain your cardiovascular fitness. As you know, you could split the 20 minutes into 2, 10-minute workouts if you do not have 20 minutes in a row. As far as resistance training is concerned, to enable you to maintain your current strength and muscle tone, the minimum is one workout per week of at least one set per body part using a challenging weight. Ideally, you should try to do two resistance training sessions per week. Once a year it is not a bad idea to skip a whole week of working out to give your body a complete rest.

More advice

By the time you finish the program you should be in great shape. Try to find a sport or activity you enjoy and try to participate on a regular basis. There are a lot of leagues you can join for different sports in your community. There are also hiking clubs, cycling clubs, and all sorts of other clubs you can join in your local community. Look into them. They are a great way to say active and fit.

I recommend weighing yourself weekly or biweekly to make sure you are maintaining your weight and you are not gaining. It is much easier, as you know, to lose one to two pounds than to lose 20 to 30 pounds. Make a promise to yourself in writing and post it where you can see it every day, that you will never let yourself go again. You have worked hard to get to the shape you are in today and you should not let it go to waste. So keep regular checks on yourself and maintenance is a breeze.

For more support, weekly updates of what's new in the weight loss and fitness field and much more, you can subscribe to my free newsletter at www.StavrosM.com.

CHAPTER 8

Conclusion

There is no secret to losing weight and getting in shape. There is no magic pill that will help you lose weight, nor will there ever be one. The truth is, it will take some effort on your part and only permanent changes in your habits will result in permanent weight loss. The fact is, to lose weight and get into shape, all you need to do is incorporate the four keys to weight loss into your life. The four keys are: resistance training, which you only need to do two to three times per week; aerobic training, which you need to do five to six times per week; proper nutrition, which basically means eating a lot more fruits and vegetables, eating less meat products and eliminating as much as possible junk food and refined food; and the last key, consistency. You have to be consistent in your efforts if you want to get results.

Any program that does not include all four keys is destined to fail. As I said before, you will have to put some effort into it. A program that promises weight loss with little or no effort is deceiving you. If it were that easy to lose weight, everybody would be thin by now. Keep in mind weight loss is not everything, being healthy is far more important. Losing weight in an unhealthy way will only harm you in the long run.

Finally, a message for anyone who says that they have no time to exercise and watch their diet: you need to reevaluate your priorities in life. WHAT IS MORE IMPORTANT THAN YOUR HEALTH?

If you follow my program, I know you will succeed not just in losing weight but also in improving your health in the process.

APPENDIX 1

Goal & Attitude Questionnaire

Name_____

Date_____

General instructions: Please answer the questions as best you can and as accurately as possible. The more thought you put into these questions, the better you will understand what stands between you and the body and health you want. This understanding will greatly improve your chances of reaching your final fitness goals.

1. What is/are your fitness goal(s)?

2. What benefits will you get from reaching the above goal(s)?

3. Have you tried to achieve the above goals before? ___Yes ___No. If yes, why didn't you reach your goal? What is holding you back? What obstacles do you have to overcome in order to achieve your goal? Please really think about all these questions, and answer them the best you can. Do not forget to list all the obstacles that stand in the way of your fitness goals, and think of possible ways to overcome these obstacles.

4. Think for a minute. What shape do you think you will be in 5, 10, or 20 years from now if you continue with your current eating & activity habits and do not change anything?

In 5 Years.

In 10 Years.

In 20 Years.

5.   Think for a minute. If you had started an exercise program last year, what shape do you think you would be in right now?

6.   On a scale from 1 to 10, 1 being not committed at all and 10 being committed 100%, how committed are you to reaching your goal(s) _____.

7.   What shape do you think you will be in next year at this time if you start an exercise program today?

APPENDIX 2 FOOD LIST

80 to 90 percent of your diet should be made up of the following foods:

Vegetables (6 to 8 servings per day)
Artichoke, Asparagus, Bell peppers, Broccoli, Brussels sprouts, Cabbage, Carrots (raw), Cauliflower, etc.

Fruits (At least 4 servings per day)
Apple, Apricot, Avocado, Banana, Berries, Cherries, Figs, Grapes, Orange, etc.

Beans & Legumes (1 to 2 servings per day)
Lentils, Chickpeas, All dried beans, Soybeans, etc.

Nuts (No more than 1 ounce per day. Raw and no salt is best)
Almonds, Brazil nuts, Chestnuts, Sunflower seeds, etc.

Best Oils (In very small amounts, 1 Tbsp per day)
Olive oil, Flaxseed oil.

Alcohol (One glass of wine per day is fine)

The following foods you should eat in limited amounts, as stated:

Whole Grain Foods (Eat 3 servings per day)
Whole wheat breads, Light sprouted bread, Rye bread, Oat meal, Whole grain low sugar cereal, etc.

Best Starch Vegetables (Do not eat more than 1 to 2 servings per day)

Potatoes, Sweet potatoes, Cooked carrots, Corn, Wild rice, Yams, etc.

All Meats and Poultry (Do not eat more than 1 to 2 servings per week)

Seafood (Eat 1 to 2 servings per week)
All small fish, Crab, Lobster, Shrimp, etc.

Dairy Foods (1 to 2 servings per day, keep it low fat)
Low fat organic milk, Low fat organic yogurt, Low fat cheese, etc.

Eggs (Organic eggs you can have 4 to 5 per week)

<u>The following foods should be avoided like the plague. (It's OK to have them as a treat once in a while) All of these foods are overly processed or too refined, high in sodium, and stripped of any nutritional value.)</u>

Refined Carbs
All precuts made with white flour and/or sugar, like white bread, cakes, ice cream, donuts, cookies, milk shakes, etc.

High Fat Proteins
All fried meats and seafood, deli meats, bacon, sausages, etc.

Beverages
Sodas, diet sodas, liquor drinks, etc.

Fats
All products that have Hydrogenated fat.

If you would like a complete list of all foods for free, just send me an email to <u>Stavros@stavrosm.com</u>, on the subject line put "Food List", and I will email you the complete list.

APPENDIX 3

HEALTHY RECIPES

If you would like more recipes, I am currently working on a new recipe book, which will be full of healthy and easy to make recipes. For more information on when it is going to be published go to www.stavrosm.com

Note: I encourage everyone to experiment with the recipes and try different vegetables, amounts, and spices to better match their personal taste. The vegetable amounts are all estimates.

Cannelini Bean Salad

Cannelini beans canned (if fresh, soak in water overnight, and then boil them until soft) 1 lb.
Scallions (chopped) 5 each.
Red & green peppers (chopped) 3 total
Olive Oil (to taste) 2 oz.
Vinegar (optional, to taste)
Salt (very little)

Mix all vegetables with beans; add olive oil and vinegar to taste.

Use as much or as little of each ingredient as you like. Go by your taste. Just make sure you do not use too much olive oil because although is good for you, too much is still fattening. This salad will stay fresh very well in the refrigerator and you can eat it cold. You can make it in bulk and have it throughout the week.

Broccoli & Red Pepper Soup

2 lbs. of *fresh or frozen broccoli*, chopped into large pieces
2 sticks of *celery*, roughly chopped.
1 large *onion*, diced
3 *garlic* cloves, chopped fine.
3 Tbsp. *dried vegetable soup mix* (such as Vogue Vege Base)
1/3 cup *brown rice* (uncooked)
3 *red bell peppers*
juice from one lemon
1 Tbsp. *vinegar*
seasonings to taste, but very little salt if any.

Step 1
In a large soup pot, combine the broccoli, celery, onion, garlic, Vege Base, and rice in 3 quarts of water. Simmer, covered.

Step 2
Cut the red peppers in half; remove the seeds and roast, half in a broiler or on a grill, skin side facing the heat source until skin side begins to blacken. Remove the peel and puree them in a blender.

Step 3
When the broccoli is soft, mash it in the pot with the rest of the vegetables using a potato masher. Add pureed red pepper to the pot. Add the lemon, vinegar, and seasonings to taste (e.g., tarragon, thyme, white or black pepper).

Artichoke Hearts with Peas

Artichoke hearts (canned) around 3 lbs. (cut them in halves)
Peas (frozen) 4 cups
Dill (chopped) handful
Scallions (chopped) 6 each
Tomato Sauce (fresh or canned) 1-½ cups
Olive oil 2 Tbsp.
Water 1 cup (as it needs it)
Salt to taste

Pepper to taste

Step 1
Sauté dill and scallions with the olive oil in a pot for 5 minutes.

Step 2
Add the frozen peas and sauté for 5 more minutes

Step 3
Add the tomato sauce, artichoke hearts, water, pepper, and very little salt and cook until artichokes get hot.

Black-Eyed Pea Salad

Black Eye Peas (if fresh, soak in water overnight, and then boil them until soft.)
Onions (chopped)
Scallions (chopped)
Tomatoes (chopped)
Romaine Lettuce (chopped thin)
Dill (chopped)
Olive Oil (to taste)
Vinegar (optional, to taste)
Salt (very little)

Mix all vegetables with peas; add olive oil and vinegar to taste.

Use as much or as little of each ingredient as you like. Go by your taste. Just make sure you do not use too much olive oil because although it is good for you, too much is still fattening. This salad will stay fresh in the refrigerator and you can eat it cold. You can make it in bulk and have it throughout the week.

Boiled Chicory salad

This great side dish is very easy to make and is very healthy for you.

It can be eaten hot or cold, so you can make it ahead of time and keep it in the refrigerator.

1 *Chicory*
Olive oil to taste
Lemon juice to taste
Very little *salt*

1. Cut the root off the chicory and wash it.
2. Boil in slightly salted water until the stem is soft, around 30 minutes.
3. Strain the water, and put it in a bowl.
4. Cut it up a little bit; add olive oil, lemon juice, and a little salt. Mix and serve.

This side dish is a great way to add vegetables to your diet. Try it.

Mediterranean Style Lima Beans

Lima beans 1 lb. bag (dry) Soak in water overnight.
Tomato sauce (canned is fine) 2 cups
Olive oil 2 Tbsp.
Onions (chopped) 1 medium
Garlic (chopped) 2 cloves
Parsley (fresh, chopped) 3 Tbsp.
Oregano to taste
Salt to taste, but use very little
Pepper to taste

Note: Make sure you have soaked the lima beans in water overnight.

Step 1 Boil beans in water with a little salt until they are soft, but not too soft, about 45 minutes.

Step 2 Sauté in the olive oil, the onions, garlic and oregano for 3 to

4 minutes, and then add the parsley, salt (very little), pepper, and tomato sauce and continue cooking for another 10 minutes.

Step 3 Once beans are done, drain them but save some of the juice, put them in an oven pan and mix in the sautéed onions, garlic, and tomato sauce mix. Add some of the saved water from the boiled beans, until beans are almost covered. Mix and put them in the oven for around 40 minutes at 350 degrees.

Peas & Corn

1 Onion chopped
Garlic 2 gloves chopped.
Mushrooms (any kind) 3 cups diced
Peeled whole tomatoes in tomato juice (canned) 1 can, chopped
Frozen peas 2 cups
Frozen corn 1 cup
Oregano to taste
Olive oil 1 Tbsp.
Black pepper to taste
Very little *salt*
Bay leaves (1 if whole, a pinch if chopped)

Step 1

Place olive oil in big pan and sauté the onions and garlic for 3 minutes.

Step 2

Add the mushrooms and sauté for 3 minutes.

Step 3

Add chopped tomatoes with the juice from the can; add the oregano, black pepper, salt, and bay leaves. Bring it to a boil.

Step 4

Once boiling, add peas and corn and cook until peas and corn are cooked, about 10 to 15 minutes. Note: leave pan uncovered.

Ratatouille

1 Eggplant (cubed)
2 Zucchini (cubed)
Green and/or red peppers 2 each (diced large)
Onions 1 large (diced)
Whole canned tomatoes 1 medium size can or 2 small ones (chopped in big chunks)
Olive oil 2 Tbsp.
Garlic 1 clove
Oregano to taste
Pepper to taste
Salt use very little

Step 1

In a pot sauté onions with the olive oil, garlic, salt, pepper, and oregano until onions are translucent.

Step 2

Add the tomatoes and cook for 5 minutes.

Step 3

Add the eggplant and cook for around 10 minutes.

Step 4

Add the zucchini, green/red peppers and cook until the vegetables are done.

Red beet salad

This makes a great side dish that very easy to make and is very healthy for you. It can be eaten hot or cold, so you could make it ahead of time and keep it in the refrigerator.

One bunch fresh *beets with their greens*
Olive oil
Vinegar

Very little *salt*

Step 1

Peel the beets and cut them in half or quarter them, depending on how big they are.

Step 2

Wash the greens and put them in a pot with the beets and fill it up with water. Boil them until you can stick a fork in them, around 30 minutes.

Step 3

Strain them well and put them in a bowl. Add little olive oil, vinegar to taste, and little salt and mix.

Spinach & Rice

Spinach, 4 lbs. If fresh, cut stems off leaves; if frozen, make sure it is defrosted.

Dill, chopped, 1 handful

Scallions (around 9) chopped

Olive oil 4 Tbsp.

Tomato juice 7 cups

Chicken stock 2 cups

Brown rice instant 1 box, 14 oz. uncooked

Oregano to taste

Salt very little

Pepper to taste

Note: Feel free to experiment with the amount of each ingredient to better suit your taste.

Step 1

In a large pot, sauté the scallions and the dill in the olive oil

Step 2

Add the oregano, salt, pepper, brown rice. Sauté for 1 minute.

Step 3

Add the tomato juice. Bring it to a boil and add the spinach. Mix and cover it. Lower the heat.

(Note: if you are using frozen spinach wait until the rice is almost cooked before adding it.)

Step 4

Keep mixing it once in the while so it will not stick. Eventually the spinach will settle down. Make sure you keep it covered as it cooks, and keep mixing it periodically.

Step 5

Cook until the rice is done.

This meal tastes even better the next day, so don't be afraid to make extra.

Spinach with Onions

1 lb. *spinach*
1 big *onion* cut in half and thinly sliced
2 cloves *garlic* finely chopped.
1 Tbsp. *olive oil*
Oregano to taste
Pepper to taste
Very little *salt*

Step 1

In a pot, sauté the onions with the garlic in the olive oil.

Step 2

Once the onions are translucent add the spinach and all the spices, and cook until spinach is done.

Tomato Salad, Greek-style

Ripe tomatoes 2 each (cut in wedges)
Green pepper 1 each (cut in half and then sliced thinly)
Red Onion ½ each (sliced thinly)
Oregano to taste
Salt to taste
Olive oil around 3 Tbsp.
Feta cheese (optional) couple of slices

Mix everything together in a bowl and serve. It tastes best if you let it sit for ½ hour before you eat.

Eggplant and Beans (Main meal)

1 *eggplant* peeled and diced
1 *onion* sliced thinly
½ *onion* finely chopped (optional)
1 *green pepper* diced
1 tbsp. *lemon juice*
3 tbsp. *ketchup*
Very little *olive oil*
2 cups *garbanzo or other beans*, cooked or canned

Step 1

Steam the eggplant for 10—12 minutes. If you do not have a steamer put eggplant in a pot with a little water and cover. Make sure you stir it often so it won't stick.

Step 2

Saute the sliced onion and pepper over a low flame in a covered skillet with very little olive oil (suggestion: wet a napkin with oil and wipe the bottom of the pan) for 6—8 minutes.

Step 3

Add the steamed eggplant, lemon juice, and ketchup in the pan with the onions and peppers and simmer uncovered for another 5 minutes.

Mix in the beans, cook until hot, and add the chopped onion right before you take it off the heat.

Mushrooms and Onion Mix (side dish)

3 cups *mushrooms* diced, use whatever mushrooms you like.
1 *onion* diced
1 to 2 tbsp. *dried vegetable soup mix* (such as Vogue Vege Base) to taste

Wet a napkin with a little olive oil and wipe the bottom of a nonstick pan. Sautee the onions and mushrooms, for 5 minutes and than add the Vege base. Cook until done.

Eggplant Patties (Main meal or side dish)

2 eggplants, peeled and sliced
3 Tbsp. balsamic vinegar
4 garlic cloves, finely chopped
1 cup vegetable stock (fat free, low sodium if possible)
1 Tbsp. finely chopped rosemary
pinch of black pepper
pinch of oregano
1 tbsp. Bragg's Liquid Aminos

Dip (optional)
½ cup fat free or 50% reduced fat mayonnaise
Garlic finely chopped, use as much as you like.

Mix the mayonnaise with the garlic.

Suggestions on how to use the dip: Do not dip the vegetables directly into the dip because you end up with too much. Instead, dip the tip of your fork in the dip and eat your vegetables with it. This way, you get the taste without overpowering the vegetables.

Step 1

Slice eggplant into 1/3 inch-thick patties.

Step 2

Mix the remaining ingredients all together all in a flat-bottom bowl.

Step 3

Wet napkin with olive oil and wipe down a nonstick baking tray or aluminum foil, creating a thin coat of oil.

Step 4

Dip the eggplant patties in the mixture for 5 seconds and then place on the oiled tray or aluminum foil.

Step 5

Bake the eggplant on the tray or sheet of aluminum foil at 350 degrees for 20—25 minutes. Mushrooms can be used instead of or in addition to the eggplant.

REFERENCES

American Council on Exercise. *Personal Trainer Manual*. San Diego, CA: American Council on Exercise, 1996.

Ballentine, R. *Diet and Nutrition—A Holistic Approach*. Honesdale, PA: The Himalayan Institute Press, 1978.

Cordain, L. *The Paleo Diet*. New York: John Wiley and Sons, 2002.

Diamond, Harvey and Marilyn. *Fit For Life*. New York: Warner Books, 1985.

Diamond, H. *The Fit for Life Solution*. St Paul, MN: Dragon Door Publications, 2002.

Faigin, R. *Natural Hormone Enhancement*. Cedar Mountain, NC: Extique Publishing, 2000.

Fuhrman, J. *Eat To Live*. New York: Little, Brown and Company, 2003.

Hofmekler, O. *The Warrior Diet*. St Paul, MN: Dragon Door Publications, 2001.

Maltz, M. *The New Psycho-Cybernetics*. New York: Prentice-Hall, 2001.

Roizen, M. and La Puma, J. *The Real Age Diet*. New York: HarperCollins, 2001.

Tilden, J.H. *Toxemia Explained*. Pomeroy WA: Health Research Books, 1960.

Wayne L. Westcott, Ph.D. and Tracy D'Arpino, B.S. LPTA. *High-Intensity Strength Training*. Health Learning, 2003.

www.ingramcontent.com/pod-product-compliance
Lightning Source LLC
Chambersburg PA
CBHW060518290526
45791CB00001B/439